Advanced Concepts in Multiple Sclerosis Nursing Care

Advanced Concepts
in

Multiple Sclerosis Nursing Care

SECOND EDITION

June Halper, MCSN, ANP, FAAN

Editor

Visit our web site at www.demosmedpub.com

LIBRARY OF CONGRESS CATALOGING-IN-PUBLICATION DATA

Advanced concepts in multiple sclerosis nursing care / June Halper, editor.—2nd ed.

p. ; cm.

Includes bibliographical references and index.

ISBN-13: 978-1-933864-15-0 (pbk. : alk. paper)

ISBN-10: 1-933864-15-X (pbk. : alk. paper)

1. Multiple sclerosis—Nursing.   I. Halper, June.

[DNLM: 1. Multiple Sclerosis—nursing.   WY 160.5 A244 2007]

RC377.A348 2007

616.8'34—dc22

2007009357

Medicine is an ever-changing science undergoing continual development. Research and clinical experience are continually expanding our knowledge, in particular our knowledge of proper treatment and drug therapy. The authors, editors, and publisher have made every effort to ensure that all information in this book is in accordance with the state of knowledge at the time of production of the book.

Nevertheless, this does not imply or express any guarantee or responsibility on the part of the authors, editors, or publisher with respect to any dosage instructions and forms of application stated in the book. Every reader should examine carefully the package inserts accompanying each drug and check with his physician or specialist whether the dosage schedules mentioned therein or the contraindications stated by the manufacturer differ from the statements made in this book. Such examination is particularly important with drugs that are either rarely used or have been newly released on the market. Every dosage schedule or every form of application used is entirely at the reader's own risk and responsibility. The editors and publisher welcome any reader to report to the publisher any discrepancies or inaccuracies noticed.

Special discounts on bulk quantities of Demos Medical Publishing books are available to corporations, professional associations, pharmaceutical companies, healthcare organizations, and other qualifying groups. For details, please contact:

Special Sales Department
Demos Medical Publishing
386 Park Avenue South, Suite 301
New York, NY 10016
Phone: 800-532-8663 or 212-683-0072
Fax: 212-683-0118
E-mail: orderdept@demosmedpub.com

Printed in Canada
07 08 09 10   5 4 3 2 1

This book is dedicated
to the memory of
Linda Morgante, RN, MSN, MSCN,

who inspired *hope* and *love*
in all whom she touched.

Contents

MULTIPLE SCLEROSIS: THE DISEASE

ADVANCED PRACTICE IN MULTIPLE SCLEROSIS NURSING

Foreword

Multiple sclerosis (MS) is a chronic, incurable, and often disabling illness that greatly impacts the lives of individuals and families. Recent
advances in MS care and treatment have made this field of healthcare both dynamic and challenging. The availability of treatments that affect the course of the
illness has increased the momentum toward disease stabilization while waiting
for a cure. The world of MS has changed from one of "wait and see" or "diagnose and adios" to one of hope and promise. Concomitantly, the role of the MS
nurse has evolved from a supportive-educative model, to a complex spectrum of
caring that still includes support and education along with skills development,
advocacy, counseling, and research. Thus, MS nurses worldwide now require
specialized skills and knowledge to meet the needs of patients and their families
who are challenged by the complexity of MS care.

Professional nurses have met theses exciting challenges by crossing oceans
and borders and networking with their peers internationally. The establishment of the International Organization of MS Nurses in 1997 reflected the new
dynamism of MS nursing. The first edition of *Advanced Concepts in Multiple
Sclerosis Nursing Care* was published to address these challenges and provide
MS nurses with new and advancing knowledge. It included advanced knowledge
on care issues from nurses involved in MS care in the United States, Canada,
and the United Kingdom. It became a valuable resource for MS nurses every-
where. Since the publication of the first edition, the world of MS has changed
significantly. The second edition reflects these changes by including chapters on
pain management, infusion therapies, complementary and alternative medicine
(CAM), expanded nursing roles, and depression in MS. The second edition can
be envisioned as an "interactive mirror" on the world of MS nurses, responding
to the changes seen in this challenging disease.

The book begins with an overview of MS by the editor and includes
current information on epidemiology, disease course, and symptom management.
She emphasizes the special needs of the severely disabled patient, and discusses
wellness-focused activities, which are often overlooked in a field focused on new
treatments. The chapter concludes with a section on empowering our patients,
which is vital in promoting self-care in an illness that constantly grabs control
from individuals.

New hope for progressive MS is discussed in a chapter written by Kathleen
Costello. This type of MS, once thought to be inevitably disabling, is now
being studied for its pathophysiology as well as for experimental treatments to
control its course. Pat Kennedy addresses the emergence of CAM in MS as a
resource to MS nurses and their patients, and she also provides an evidence-

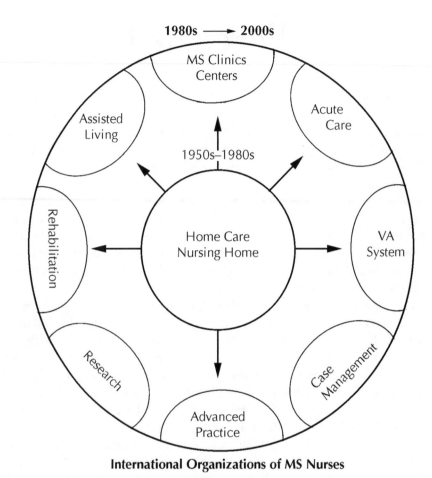

International Organizations of MS Nurses

Evolution of multiples sclerosis nursing.

based approach to the use of CAM for patient and family education. Linda Morgante not only writes about the responsibilities of the nurse research coordinator, which is vital to facilitating the collection of clinical data, but also closes the book with the hope that the uncertainty of MS will be changed during the coming decade.

The 21st century has brought with it the impetus for evidence-based practice, particularly for nurses who are in areas of advanced practice. Dr. Elsie Gulick, herself an internationally recognized nursing researcher, takes us through the research process and clarifies the steps involved in data collection, statistical analysis, and dissemination to the nursing community.

The complexities of MS care and the need for case management are updated from the first edition and adapted into an advanced practice model by

June Halper, who has also provided a new chapter dealing with existing and emerging intravenous therapies. Marie Namey, an MS nurse expert, elaborates on issues related to promoting adherence to complex protocols, as MS care becomes more sophisticated, complicated, and self-directed. Linda Lehman and Dr. Mary Ann Picone (with the input of June Halper) elaborate on the pathophysiology and management of pulmonary complications in MS. This complication is often overlooked in symptom management protocols, and yet it is the leading cause of mortality and the most frequent reason for hospital admissions. Case studies are used to outline the protocol of management for this complication.

Nursing management of complex issues in MS include cognitive impairment, pain, depression, and spasticity. The chapter on spasticity from the first edition has been updated for our readers. The management of this complex problem is addressed by three nurse contributors, focusing on the strategies and challenges for dealing with the symptom both pharmacologically and nonpharmacologically. In particular, they examine the role of oral medications and rehabilitation, both of which are enhanced by new and emerging technology. Innovations in pump design and options for self-management are described and are applicable both in North America and on the European continent. Dr. Colleen Miller discusses the crucial role of the nurse in recognizing and treating cognitive impairment with new information about this complex topic. Chapters dealing with the invisible symptoms of pain and depression have been added to the second edition by Heidi Maloni and June Halper to expand the nursing skills and knowledge required in this new era of care and caring.

The second edition of *Advanced Concepts in Multiple Sclerosis Nursing Care* is a collaborative effort of MS nurse experts from several countries. It is representative of the current trend of MS nursing, which is becoming more advanced, specialized, and complex. It also reflects the emerging role of MS nurses who are influencing care internationally. It is a valuable resource for nurses working in a variety of healthcare settings all over the world. Once again, June Halper has masterminded a valuable addition to the growing collection of MS nursing literature.

Colleen Harris, RN, MN, MSCN
Past-President
International Organization of MS Nurses (IOMSN)

Preface

This is the second edition of a book that seeks to provide an in-depth, multidimensional, systems approach to the complex care of multiple sclerosis (MS) patients. While its primary focus is on nursing, all healthcare professionals who provide MS care will find it valuable. The book is organized into sections addressing the nature of the disease, advanced practice concepts and their application to MS management, advanced symptom management, and a comprehensive nursing care plan for MS. It will provide the reader with an updated view of MS along with a greater understanding of its lifelong impact.

Nursing care has advanced from a "support service" to a partnership in the disease-management approach to MS care. The nurse plays a vital role as an educator, care provider, and advocate for patients and families affected by the disease, and does so in a wide variety of practice settings.

During the past several years, the entire concept of caring for people with MS has evolved to be more evidence based and protocol driven as we attempt to promote the highest standards of care and quality of life. The complexity of MS and the variable needs of patients and their families challenge nurses to reassess and reaffirm their commitment to long-term management. The themes of this work are the concepts of empowerment and hope, driving forces for patients, families, and their nursing partners.

Contributors to the second edition of *Advanced Concepts in Multiple Sclerosis Nursing Care* are nurse clinicians and researchers who work in geographically diverse practice settings throughout North America and the United Kingdom. Many of the authors participate in MS research in addition to their traditional nursing roles.

I anticipate that the second edition of *Advanced Concepts in Multiple Sclerosis Nursing Care* will assist nurses and other healthcare professionals who care for MS patients and their families to navigate the complex world of MS. I hope that it will provide nurses with tools and strategies to improve the lives of those affected by MS and to reinforce the role of the nurse in this challenging neurologic illness. It can also be thought to represent a comprehensive model for the care of other chronic diseases, utilizing newer concepts in nursing care and research. In this regard, I hope that this book will be considered an addition to nursing literature and become a valuable adjunct to teaching programs in nursing schools and in postgraduate nursing education.

June Halper, MSCN, ANP, FAAN
Editor

Acknowledgments

A special note of appreciation to my terrific family during the development of this book, and always—Michael, Matthew, and Julie Halper, and Ernie, Lee, and Hallie Wilson; and with love and remembrance of my late husband, Morris Halper, MD; to my patients, the families who are my heroes and heroines; and to the late Connie Boardman, who was my "iron butterfly."

Contributors

Kathleen Costello, RN, MS, CRNP, MSCN Clinical Director, Maryland MS Center, University of Maryland, Baltimore, Maryland.

Elsie E. Gulick, PhD, RN, FAAN Professor Emeritus, College of Nursing, Rutgers, The State University of New Jersey, Newark, New Jersey.

June Halper, MSCN, ANP, FAAN Executive Director, Multiple Sclerosis Comprehensive Care Center, Holy Name Hospital, Teaneck, New Jersey.

Colleen Harris, RN, NP, MSCN Nurse Practitioner, Calgary Multiple Sclerosis Clinic, Foothills Hospital, Calgary, Alberta, Canada.

Louise Jarrett, RGN, BA Hons Clinical Nurse Specialist Spasticity Management, The National Hospital for Neurology and Neurosurgery, Queen Square, London, United Kingdom.

Jane Johnson, BEd, RN, MSc Rehabilitation Clinical Development Nurse Manager, Regional Rehabilitation Unit, Northwick Park Hospital, Harrow, Middlesex, United Kingdom.

Patricia M. Kennedy, RN, CNP, MSCN Nurse Practitioner, Rocky Mountain Multiple Sclerosis Center, Englewood, Colorado.

Linda Lehman, MSN, FNP Risk Management Coordinator, Mt. Sinai Medical Center, New York, New York.

Heidi Maloni, PhDc, RN, APRN, BC-ANP, CNRN, MSCN Patient Care and Research Coordinator, Multiple Sclerosis Center of Excellence East, Veterans Affairs Medical Center, Washington, DC.

Colleen Murphy Miller, RN, CNS, NP, DNS William C. Baird Multiple Sclerosis Research Center, Buffalo General Hospital, and Department of Neurology, State University of New York at Buffalo, School of Medicine and Biomedical Sciences, Buffalo, New York.

Linda A. Morgante, MSN, RN, CRRN, MSCN Advanced Practice Nurse and Assistant Professor, Department of Nursing, Saint Joseph's College, Brooklyn, New York.

Marie A. Namey, RN, MSN, MSCN Clinical Nurse Specialist, The Edward J. and Louise E. Mellen Center for Multiple Sclerosis, The Cleveland Clinic, Cleveland, Ohio.

Mary Ann Picone, MD   Medical Director,   Multiple Sclerosis Comprehensive Care Center, Holy Name Hospital, Teaneck, New Jersey.

Bernadette Porter, RGN, CNS-MS   Consultant Nurse Multiple Sclerosis, The National Hospital for Neurology and Neurosurgery, Queen Square, London, United Kingdom.

Amy Perrin Ross, RN, MSN, CNRN   Neuroscience Program Coordinator, Loyola University Medical Center, Maywood, Illinois.

CHAPTER 1

The Nature of Multiple Sclerosis

June Halper

Multiple sclerosis (MS) is a chronic disease of the central nervous system (CNS) that most often affects young adults in the prime of their lives. Its management has evolved from a disease that was difficult to diagnose and treat in the early part of the 20th century to a condition that is better understood and treated in the 21st century. It is diagnosed almost four times as frequently in women as in men and, second to stroke, it is the most common neurologic disorder in North America. Most patients initially experience a relapsing-remitting course in which exacerbations are followed by periods of remission. The disease often converts to a progressive course, in which chronic problems and disability gradually accumulate and acute relapses no longer occur. Common symptoms include but are not limited to fatigue, reduced mobility, visual abnormalities, bladder and bowel dysfunction, sensory problems, sexual dysfunction, cognitive loss, and emotional disturbance (1).

Overview

Originally, MS was defined as relapsing-remitting and chronic-progressive. These classifications made it difficult to study the disease and to group patients into like categories. To address this problem, an international survey was conducted

Types and Courses of MS

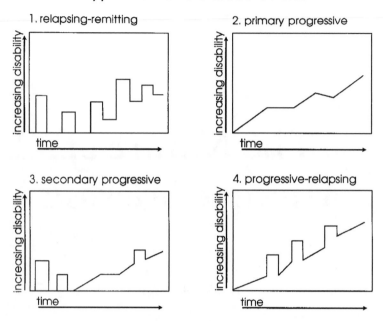

FIGURE 1-1

1. Relapsing-remitting (RR) MS is characterized by clearly defined acute attacks with full recovery or with sequelae and residual deficit upon recovery. Periods between disease relapses are characterized by lack of disease progression. **2.** Primary-progressive (PP) MS is characterized by disease showing progression of disability from onset, without plateaus or remissions, or with occasional plateaus and temporary minor improvements. **3.** Secondary-progressive (SP) MS begins with an initial RR course, followed by progression of variable rate, which may also include occasional relapses and minor remissions. **4.** Progressive-relapsing (PR) MS shows progression from onset but with clear acute relapses, with or without recovery.

in 1996 to standardize the terminology used to describe the clinical course of MS. This led to four major classifications of the disease (2), as shown in Figure 1-1.

- *Relapsing-remitting* MS has clearly defined relapses followed by periods that are characterized by a lack of disease progression and by stabilization between attacks.
- *Secondary-progressive* MS is defined as an initial relapsing-remitting course followed by progression with or without occasional relapses, minor remissions, and plateaus.
- *Primary-progressive* disease is demonstrated by a nearly continuously worsening disease course that may be interrupted by occasional plateaus and temporary minor improvements.

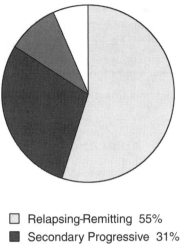

☐ Relapsing-Remitting 55%
■ Secondary Progressive 31%
■ Primary Progressive 9%
☐ Progressive-Relapsing 5%

FIGURE 1-2

Pattern of disease by type across a representative population in New York State (4).

- *Progressive-relapsing* MS is progressive disease from the outset, with clear acute relapses with or without recovery.

As noted by Coyle (3), relapsing MS is the characteristic onset in 85% of patients, primary progressive in 10%, and progressive relapsing in 5%. Approximately 75% of people with relapsing MS change to a secondary progressive course after some years, and the overall pattern of disease resembles that shown in Figure 1-2, which provides one perspective of disease course distribution. Progressive patients tend to be male and older, and up to 30% stabilize over time (3).

An *exacerbation* is defined as a new onset of neurologic symptoms lasting 24 to 48 hours without metabolic etiology. Ninety-six percent of patients recover from the first attack, with subsequent episodes occurring from less than 1 year to within 5 years. Attacks may diminish over time as patients begin a secondary progressive course, usually 6 to 10 years into their disease (3).

The cause of MS is not known, although it is suspected to be the result of an immunologic response to an environmental trigger commonly related to viral infections in genetically susceptible individuals. Several viruses have been detected in people with MS, but no single virus has been identified as a causative agent. It is possible that more than one virus is capable of triggering this response (5). For decades, MS has been defined as a demyelinating disease with inflammation and subsequent repair. More recent evidence points to a more ominous picture, with neurodegeneration (axonal destruction) resulting in permanent and irreversible damage (6). This new understanding of the nature of the disease results in a broader implication that impels early diagnosis and prompt disease management.

The average life span of a person with MS is generally not substantially decreased; it is 2 years less than average (3). The cost of MS over a lifetime has been estimated at $2.2 million (1994 dollars); relapsing MS approximately $30,000 per year; and progressive disease approximately $50,000 per year (7).

Epidemiology

Multiple sclerosis is the most frequently acquired neurologic disease in young adults; it affects proportionally mostly Caucasians (90%). It is unusual for people in Africa and Asia to be diagnosed (9). There is approximately a 40% incidence in African Americans, with a potential genetic etiology. High-risk areas include the northern United States and Canada, northern Europe, southern Australia, and New Zealand (8). The age of onset is usually within a few years of puberty, with 30 years being the approximate average age. More than 70% of individuals with MS are women, a factor that is unexplained in the literature (3) except for the fact that most autoimmune diseases are more common in women.

Diagnosis

The diagnosis of MS is based on clinical criteria established by Schumacher in 1965 and redefined by Poser and coworkers in 1983 (10). In the early 1990s McDonald et al modernized the diagnostic criteria to include technological advances such as MRI, evoked potentials, and cerebrospinal fluid analysis (11). The McDonald criteria (Table 1-1) were updated recently to include more MRI parameters to facilitate a more prompt and accurate diagnosis. Ultimately, the diagnosis remains a clinical one because, although laboratory tests may be supportive, they are not clearly definitive without the clinical expertise to confirm MS and rule out other confounding condition. Cranial magnetic resonance imaging (MRI) is eventually abnormal in 90 to 95% of patients, but the test lacks the specificity to state that the lesions are definitely caused by MS (8). Figure 1-3 shows the laboratory workup used in the diagnostic process, and Table 1-2 summarizes prognostic indicators.

Treatment of Acute Exacerbations: Assessment and Treatment

The treatment of acute exacerbations is based on the severity of the attack. Intravenous corticosteroids have shown to shorten the duration of significant

TABLE 1-1
Diagnosis—criteria

Clinical attacks	Objective lesions	Additional requirements
≥2	≥2	• None, clinical evidence will suffice
≥2	1	• Dissemination in space by MRI OR +ve CSF + ≥2 MRI lesions OR further clinical attack involving different site
1	≥2	• Dissemination in time by MRI OR 2nd clinical attack
1 (mono-symptomatic)	1	• Dissemination in space by MRI OR +ve CSF + ≥2 MRI lesions AND • Dissemination in time by MRI or 2nd clinical attack
0 (progression from onset)	1	• +ve CSF AND • Dissemination in space by MRI evidence of multiple brain and/or cord lesions OR +ve VEP with multiple MRI lesions AND • Dissemination in time by MRI or continued progression for 1 year

McDonald WI, et al. *Ann Neurol.* 2001;50:121–127.

attacks; sensory attacks are usually self-limited and may not be treated pharmaceutically (1). Intravenous (IV) therapy is usually provided with methyl-prednisolone, 1 to 3 g daily for 3 to 5 days. This may or may not be followed by an oral taper with oral corticosteroids (dexamethasone, methylprednilosone, prednisoione or prednisone. ACTH may be a treatment option while some prescribers opt for oral corticosteroids. (for more a extensive discussion see chapter 5 on relapses management by Harris). Long-term administration of corticosteroids is not recommended because of their significant toxic effects and the lack of evidence of long-term benefit. Side effects include susceptibility to opportunistic infections, hypertension, cataracts, muscle wasting, osteoporosis, and diabetes (8). Adrenocorticotropic hormone (ACTH) was a treatment for acute relapses during the mid-20th century (12). It fell out of favor for many years, but has returned as a treatment option during the early part of the 21st century. Dosing ranges from 80 units for 5 days either intramuscularly (IM) or subcutaneously (SC), or 80 units for 5 days; 40 units for 5 days, and 20 units for 5days either SC or IM. Studies are under way to determine dosing, frequency, and type of parenteral delivery (IM versus SC).

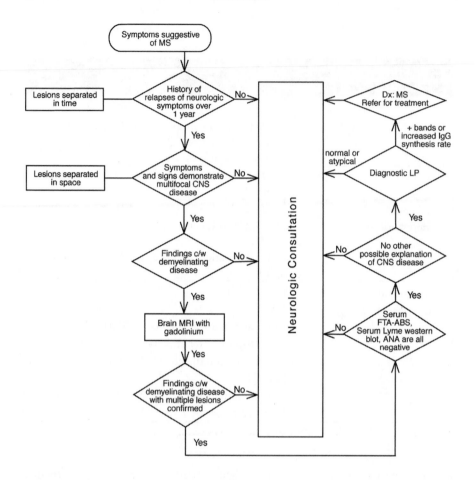

FIGURE 1-3

The differential diagnosis of multiple sclerosis. Reprinted with permission from Vollmer T. Multiple sclerosis: The Disease and Its Diagnosis. In: van den Noort S, Holland NJ , eds. *Multiple sclerosis in clinical practice*. New York: Demos Medical Publishing, 1999.

Disease Modifying Therapies

During the past decade, a number of agents have become treatment options for reducing exacerbations, modifying the disease course, and having an impact on disability. These include interferon beta-1b (Betaseron), interferon beta-1a (Avonex and Rebif), and glatiramer acetate (Copaxone). The interferons are immunomodulating agents that are injected SC every other day, IM weekly, and three times a week, respectively (9). Copaxone's components mimic myelin basic protein, which competes for binding sites and possibly interrupts the inflammatory cascade in the demyelination process (12).

TABLE 1-2

Clinical Factors with Prognostic Value in Multiple Sclerosis

Favorable	Unfavorable
Younger age at onset	Older age at onset
Female	Male
Normal MRI at presentation	High lesion load on MRI at presentation
Complete recovery from first relapse	Lack of recovery from first relapse
Low relapse rate	High relapse rate Early cerebellar involvement
Long interval to second relapse	Short interval to second relapse
Low disability at 2 and 4 years	Early development of mild disability Insidious motor onset

From Dr. P. K. Coyle, personal communication.

Side effects of the interferons include flu-like reactions, spasticity, injection site reactions with injectable therapies (interferon beta-1b and glatiramer acetate), and altered hematologic and hepatic profiles with the interferons. Nursing strategies to reduce side effects include encouraging the patient to warm the solution to room temperature (perhaps body temperature); dose titration of interferon therapy upon initiation of treatment; and personalized information and education to reduce anxiety and sustain hope. Systemic side effects with the interferons can be minimized by timing the administration of the drug in the evening, premedicating with nonsteroidal anti-inflammatory drugs (NSAIDs), rotating injection sites, and using sterile technique (9). Copaxone may rarely result in a mild, transient systemic reaction that resolves spontaneously over a short period of time (11). There is no need to monitor blood work with Copaxone, but interferon therapy requires regular blood work to monitor complete blood count and liver function. Natalizumba (Tysabri®) was approved for relapsing MS in 2004, withdrawn in 2005 due to safety concerns, and reintroduced in 2006. It is recommended for use in relapsing patients who have not responded to injectable therapies or who are intolerant of side-effects. It is monitored by an FDA-mandated safety program and is infused every four weeks. Chapter 4 discusses the role of the nurse in injectable and infusible therapies.

The Role of Nursing

The nurse is a key member of a team of healthcare professionals tending to the patient with MS and the family. Day-to-day contact, knowledge, and awareness of critical issues in MS make the nurse well suited to make certain patient evaluations. In addition, the nurse often serves as a liaison between the patient, family, and healthcare providers, and can be instrumental in the design of a comprehensive treatment plan for the patient (13).

The first type of evaluation commonly made by the nurse is an assessment of the patient's physiologic status and needs. A nurse is perhaps the best person to observe subtle changes in bowel and bladder function, mobility, swallowing, vision, and skin integrity. Keen observation makes it possible to treat such symptoms promptly, sometimes preventing the development of serious complications.

Because people with MS are at increased risk for depression and suicide, it is also important for the nurse to pay close attention to their psychological state and needs (14). Changes in behavior, expressions of helplessness, hopelessness, anger, sadness, and suicidal statements should be noted and reported to other members of the healthcare team. A study of suicide among people with MS found that those who had committed suicide were more likely to be male, unemployed, experiencing financial stress, more severely disabled, in a progressive phase of the disease, experiencing unendurable psychic pain, withdrawn, and isolated from a support network (15).

Nurses are usually able to assess the relationship between the patient and his or her care partners and can often determine whether the care partners are helping or hindering the process. The educational level of family members (how much they understand about the disease process, symptoms, and treatments) can also be evaluated. The patient and family should understand that two-thirds of all people with MS do not become severely disabled, and that most people with MS live a relatively normal life. Any gaps in knowledge can be filled in with readings, support groups, or individual educational sessions with the nurse as that of the care partners. Success in the management of MS depends on the attitude and outlook of the patient and his or her support network (16) and their outlook on MS in relation to the future.

Nurses who care for people with MS should be aware of specific concerns about their disease. Patients may ask "What will happen to me and my family?" "Can I continue working?" "How disabled will I become?" Preexisting insecurities often become exaggerated. Nurses must assist these patients to become educated about their disease and suggested treatments. Patients should be encouraged to seek counseling to overcome depression and possibly to affiliate with support groups that provide understanding and empathyx (17).

Since MS usually strikes during the productive years of life, issues related to employment can be a prominent concern. It is estimated that 25% of those with MS are working ten years after diagnosis but are at least 25% who desire to return to the work force. Fatigue and other symptoms and a progressive disease course impose major obstacles to sustained employment and promote hopeless feelings about the future. Nurses, social workers, and physicians can be supportive in encouraging a patient to continue to work, if possible. Since working and productivity are important to a person's quality of life this goal should be kept in mind throughout the spectrum of caring. Finding a job that is not physically demanding, staggering work hours, napping, and working from home are models one can use to assist people with MS to remain in the work force. Those who are no longer able to work should be encouraged to find volunteer, community, and educational activities appropriate to physical and mental function. Adaptive devices such as scooters, voice-activated computers, and visual aids can assist patients remain active and productive (18).

People with MS may worry about gender-specific issues such as sexual function; parenting; hormonally mediated events (menstruation, pregnancy, and menopause) and their roles and responsibilities as men and women. Nurses assist patients by educating them about their symptoms and Frank discussions and open dialogues about private concerns such as intercourse, erectile dysfunction, vaginal dryness, and diminished libido foster trust and a therapeutic relationship. Medications, counseling and education have proven to overcome changes wrought by MS (19).

With the possible exception of men with retrograde ejaculation, fertility is not impaired in people with MS. There is a lower risk of exacerbations during pregnancy and a higher risk 3 to 8 months postpartum. The patient and partner must consider all aspects of parenting before deciding whether to start or expand a family. It is very likely that many couples would welcome information about their choices and options. A nurse should encourage couples to be realistic about problems associated with the disease; to evaluate their emotional, financial, and family support surroundings; to assess their flexibility with parenting roles; and to think beyond the initial stages of infancy. Couples should also be made aware of the resources available to them, including educational materials, family therapists, and support groups (20).

A parent's diagnosis of MS can be difficult for young children. A child's sense of security can be threatened by the disability of the parent. In addition, a child may have to shift roles and assume a caregiver role for the parent. Although a parent with MS should avoid giving elaborate details of symptoms and disability, children become more anxious when they sense that the truth is being kept from them. Parents should give age-appropriate answers to questions. Family strain may also result from progressive or unpredictable disease. Family counseling can alleviate the burden of caregiving by affording spouses and partners the opportunity to air their concerns and develop strategies for coping (21).

The nurse plays a vital role as an educator, counselor, and advocate for patients and their family members. It is important to encourage those affected by MS to move out of a passive role and assume a proactive stance about the disease. By becoming educated, the patient is more likely to feel a sense of empowerment, acceptance, and well-being. The nurse can assist in this process by referring patients to literature, newsletters, and short-term orientation groups and by explaining the disease process, symptoms, tests, and technical terms.

It is important for a nurse to help establish reasonable expectations for proposed treatments, to educate patients in self-care and wellness, and to explain side effects. A nurse's support, advice, education, and expertise can do much to assist patients to see MS as a manageable part of their lives rather than an uncontrollable and unpredictable condition. Multiple sclerosis provides nurses with unique opportunities to promote maximal functional and wellness in their patients and their families. These interventions can promote a good quality of life in those who have been affected by this difficult and challenging disease (22).

Pediatric MS

During the past decade there has been increasing interest in pediatric MS. Modeled after the program for children in Toronto, Canada, several pediatric MS units have been founded in the United States with specialized care support and research opportunities for children and their parents. Numerous MS nurses have been involved and extremely valuable in these new and expanding programs.

Managing Difficult Symptoms of Multiple Sclerosis

Primary symptoms in MS are the direct result of demyelination in the CNS. They primarily include weakness, fatigue, tremor, pain, bladder and bowel dysfunction, paralysis, spasticity, visual changes, and diminished sexual function, including impotence in men (23). *Secondary symptoms* are complications caused by the underlying impairment. These include falls, injury, reduced activities of daily living, lack of sleep, urinary tract infection (UTI), incontinence of bowel and bladder, skin breakdown, contractures, problems with the environment (physical barriers that preclude mobility; safety hazards), and diminished opportunities for intimacy. *Tertiary symptoms* are psychosocial or vocational problems that occur when primary and secondary symptoms are not treated and become an overwhelming part of the patient's life. They include loss of job; shift in roles; divorce; loss of financial, social, vocational, and environmental mobility; the stigma of disability; and reactive depression (24).

By taking measures to alleviate primary symptoms, the incidence of secondary and tertiary symptoms may be reduced dramatically. However, it is important to note that the greatest impact on the patient's quality of life is made by measures to reduce disability and handicap despite the persistence of primary symptoms. It is equally important to point out to patients that, while disease modifying agents may impact disability and disease progression, symptoms may persist and should be addressed individually and dynamically. Although not all frequently encountered symptoms of MS are fully discussed in this book, more comprehensive information may be found in *Multiple Sclerosis: Key Issues in Nursing Management* (22).

Fatigue

Fatigue is a common symptom in MS, whatever the patient's physical status. Typically, a patient becomes tired after exercise or as the day progresses. Some people may also complain of sudden episodes of fatigue or awakening with fatigue despite a full night's sleep. Effective energy-conserving techniques include scheduling regular rest periods or short naps, performing moderate exercises, and using assistive devices such as a motorized scooter. Medications for fatigue include modafinil (Provigil), 100 mg to 200 mg every day; amantadine (Symmetrel), 100 mg twice a day; and fluoxetine (Prozac), 10 mg every day. Depression can be a cause of fatigue, and treatments such as counseling and a supportive social environment can be therapeutic in combating this problem (24). New research in MS points to the role of sleep disruption that may result in ongoing fatigue. Some of the many factors that affect sleep quality include pain, nocturia, depression, and side effects of medications. Because of the potential for sleep disturbance to lead to daytime somnolence, increased fatigue, dangerous respiratory events, and reduce quality of life, MS clinicians must be prepared to identify and treat patients sleep disorders (24, 25).

Vertigo

Vertigo may occur either intermittently or chronically. Antihistamines and anxiolytic drugs such as diazepam (Valium), clonazepam (Klonopin), and oxazepam (Serax) are commonly used along with rehabilitation techniques such as *habituation* programs. Habituation exercises are used by physical therapists to assist patients to tolerate vertigo and circumvent its effect. Head rotation and other movements may reduce the perception of this disturbing symptom (234).

Bladder and Bowel Dysfunction

Many patients with MS experience some type of bladder problem during the course of the disease. Symptoms may include urinary urgency, frequency, incontinence, nocturia, and frequent UTI. Bladder dysfunction is managed by obtaining a careful history, ruling out a UTI through a urinalysis and culture and sensitivity test, and obtaining a postvoid residual (PVR) volume of urine. This will help determine whether the patient has a storage or an emptying problem, or a bladder that combines the two DESD (25).

Treatment of a bladder that cannot store urine (one that has a PVR volume of less than 100 mL) consists of anticholinergic agents such as oxybutynin (Ditropan or Ditropan XL), hyoscyamine sulfate (Levsin), solifenacin succinate (Vesicare), darifenacin (Enablex), oxybutynin transdermal (Oxytrol) and propantheline bromide (Pro-Banthine), or antimuscarinic medications such as tolterodine tartrate (Detrol or Detrol LA). It is advisable for patients to reduce or avoid diuretic substances such as caffeine and aspartame and to maintain a regular schedule for bladder emptying. The bladder that fails to empty is treated with intermittent catheterization by either the patient or a care partner or by the use of an indwelling catheter. Treatment of combined dysfunction, which encompasses both failure to store and failure to empty, usually consists of anticholinergic agents along with a catheterization program (27).

Bowel dysfunction can manifest as constipation, involuntary bowel, or diarrhea. For constipation, an adequate intake of fluids and fiber, a bowel program that consists of regular and adequate time for evacuation, and stool softeners usually are effective in the management of this problem. Oral and rectal stimulants can also be used occasionally under nursing supervision, but the frequent use of enemas and harsh laxatives should be minimized. Diarrhea is usually a secondary effect of overuse of laxatives or stool softener or may occur with severe constipation when there is a leakage of intestinal contents around stool impaction. Diarrhea may be treated with remedies that reduce gastrointestinal mobility and fluid loss. Bulk-forming supplements may be beneficial (25).

Sensory Symptoms

Sensory symptoms such as pain, numbness, burning, and tingling may be a source of great concern to the patient. Symptomatic relief can be achieved by treatment with phenytoin (Dilantin), gabapentin (Neurontin), pregabalin (Lyrica), duloxetine (Cymbalta), tizanidine (Zanaflex), amitriptyline (Elavil), or carbamazepine (Tegretol). Avoidance of noxious stimuli such as tight clothing or irritating fabrics, investigation for underlying infections, and neurologic evaluation for exacerbations are recommended for these symptoms, especially if they occur acutely (24).

Pain may be either a primary symptom or the result of the disability associated with the disease. Tension headache or migraine headache may be primary symptoms, and are usually treated with prescription NSAIDs; triptan medications such as sumatriptan (Imitrex), rizatriptan (Maxalt), eletriptan (Relpax), or other drugs in this class; bupropion HCI (Zyban); or with over-the-counter pain relievers. Retro-orbital pain resulting from optic neuritis, an exacerbation of MS, is treated with steroids, usually given intravenously over 3 to 5 days. Trigeminal neuralgia or *tic douloureux* is a sharp facial pain associated with MS. Treatment consists of oral medication such as gabapentin (Neurontin), carbamazepine (Tegretol), phenytoin (Dilantin), pregabalin (Lyrica), duloxetine (Cymbalta), and baclofen (Lioresal). Botox injections may result in sustained benefit, but patients may require retreatment. Intractable neuralgia can be treated noninvasively with gamma knife irradiation or surgically with percutaneous rhizotomy, in which the sensory root fibers of the trigeminal nerve are severed. *Dysesthetic* pain, or burning or electric shock sensation in the extremities or trunk, can be alleviated with the same medications used for trigeminal neuralgia or application of capsaic acid cream (27).

Secondary pain is usually musculoskeletal in nature and is the consequence of poor posture or balance. Patients who ambulate with an inappropriate assistive device, sit or rest with poor posture and body alignment, or fall frequently may experience this symptom. Treatment consists of moderate moist heat, massage, physical therapy for appropriate seating and body alignment, pain relievers, NSAIDs, and correction of the underlying problems (23). The emergence of pain centers throughout the world has permitted significant improvement in this disabling symptom when the aforementioned measures fail or are unsatisfactory.

Facing Disease Progression

Approximately 85% of people diagnosed with MS initially experience a relapsing remitting course (1). Natural history studies indicate approximately 75% convert to a secondary progressive course over time (8). The period of worsening, which is referred to as *disease transition*, is a unique and taxing period for patients, families, and healthcare providers. In addition to more frequent exacerbations, there are more symptomatic complaints, ongoing functional decline, and a more intense need for care and reassurance. In addition to pharmacotherapeutic interventions, patients may require nonpharmacotherapeutic measures such as rehabilitation, counseling, vocational reassessment and retraining, and assistance with access to home programs and community supports. At this time, the MS team must develop and sustain a dynamic plan of care to address the variable and frightening transition. (see Chapter 2 by Costello)

The Special Needs of Those with Advanced Multiple Sclerosis

Severely disabled patients with MS may need intensive nursing care and monitoring. The family and care providers and/or partners have increased needs for concrete support (respite care, home care services) and education (27).

Patients with dysphagia must be taught dietary modifications that will prevent aspiration and nutritional deficits. Thickened fluid, soft food, and special feeding techniques must be initiated and taught to care partners and/or providers. Speech-language pathologists are particularly helpful with feeding strategies taught to the care team during this time. In more advanced disability, the person who is unable to swallow safely may be fed through a feeding tube (percutaneous endoscopic gastrostomy [PEG]) (27).

Skin care is another particular concern for the severely disabled and less mobile person. Pressure sores often occur over bony prominences, such as on the sacrum, ankles, elbows, and on pressure points, such as the heel. Signs to look for are reddened or blistered areas or blackened soft areas. Recommended measures to prevent pressure sores include the use of wheelchair cushions, wheelchairs that are well fitted to the patient, assistive devices (e.g., side rails, a trapeze, etc.) to promote repositioning, and frequent skin care measures and inspection (27).

If skin breakdown does occur, prompt wound care is recommended, with utilization of protocols that have been described and published in the nursing literature. Assessment tools such as the Braden and Norton scales are excellent resources to promptly identify high-risk patients with the goal of preventing skin breakdown (27).

The Wellness Model in Multiple Sclerosis

The variable pattern of MS, along with the uncertainty and loss of control resulting from this type of the disease, impels the nurse to respond with dynamic, individualized interventions that reflect each patient's needs. In a disease that has no cure, the patient and family must assume ongoing responsibility for healthcare and self-monitoring. Clark's Wellness Model has implications for the nursing process in this disease (28). It is a collaboration between the patient and the nurse, a positive striving toward self-awareness and self-responsibility. Clark defines the "wellness" process as unique to the individual, such that a person can be ill and still have a deep appreciation for the joy of living and a purpose in life (28).

Wellness Activities in Multiple Sclerosis

Pharmaceutical remedies are not the only way to manage MS. The proper combination of rest and physical activity is an integral part of good health and wellness. Patients can effectively conserve their strength by scheduling activities during periods when energy levels are high and by taking regular rest periods. Exercise is essential to maintain muscle strength and tone and joint mobility. Based on the work of Petajan (23) and others, it is becoming increasingly evident that physical conditioning is a vital component of wellness for people with MS. Swimming is an ideal activity because cool water prevents elevation of body temperature and buoyancy facilitates movement. Other highly recommended physical activities include stretching exercises, yoga, and t'ai chi. Heat and humidity can intensify symptoms, so it is recommended that the patient's living and working environment be kept as cool as possible, preferably with air-conditioning. Should a patient have a fever, it is important to reduce body temperature and treat the underlying cause as promptly as possible (23).

A balanced diet tailored to individual taste and the patient's physical capabilities can promote wellness. On the other hand, poor nutrition can make a patient more prone to infection and complications resulting from inadequate food and fluid intake. It also is important to note that maintenance of proper body weight is desirable for a variety of reasons: skin turgor, prevention of skin breakdown, and prevention of complications caused by being underweight or overweight. Adequate fluids, fruits, vegetables, and fiber can prevent constipation, a common complaint in MS. Cranberry juice or prune juice can increase urinary acidity and act as a bacteriostatic agent; orange juice and grapefruit juice have the opposite effect, and their intake should be limited.

Symptomatic management and wellness activities are ongoing needs in MS. The dynamic nature of the disease demands creativity and flexibility on the part of the patient, family, and healthcare provider. With these goals in mind, nurses are and can be key players to empower patients to take on new roles and responsibilities in their disease management and with the lifetime challenges imposed by multiple sclerosis.

Empowerment

The term *empowerment* has been used frequently during the past decade to depict a variety of social movements, particularly those that address the concerns of disenfranchised groups such as minority populations, the disabled, and women. The term *empower* connotes the ability to enable or authorize appropriate activities for underserved segments of the population (29).

Multiple sclerosis is a chronic disability that changes an individual's life and self-perception (30). With the assistance of significant others and healthcare professionals, a person with MS must manage symptoms, implement and adhere to prescribed treatments, and make modifications in lifestyle and behaviors to adapt to his or her illness (29). It has been theorized that a person needs unifying beliefs, religious or otherwise, to effectively deal with the uncertainty of MS and to become more positive and proactive (30).

Empowerment in MS can also be defined as consisting of self-direction with a strong underpinning of hope, a significant factor in coping and adaptation, especially having a consistent spiritual hope (30). Those with spiritual hope have been found to be better able to set goals and have stronger relationships and supports (30). Thus, empowerment and hope are related concepts. Empowerment enables the recognition and mobilization of strengths and resources. It involves knowledge, skill development, coping, mastery over the environment, and flexibility. Empowerment helps a person validate his or her sense of self-worth and value to others—friends, family, healthcare providers, and those in the community at large. Empowerment is a long-term process, one that depends on individual and family motivation and energy, social and emotional support, coping strategies, education, and community and personal resources. With empowerment, one may feel hopeful and capable; the opposite feeling is one of powerlessness.

Empowerment flows from interpersonal or spiritual sources, systems that are found in daily life—family support, professional activities, structured or unstructured support programs, and educational activities. Systems that are patient-driven empower the user of that system, whereas those that are externally imposed tend to weaken the user. For example, support groups that offer mutual aid call attention to the inherent sense of empowerment that accompanies the self-healing process (31). This form of support is a tool that a member of the group can take away, even after group termination. In contrast, externally imposed protocols with no insight into patient needs and mores tend to be less successful. This phenomenon is seen in many situations in which personal values, lifestyle, and quality-of-life issues are not considered when protocols are initiated (32).

It has been theorized that empowerment may be likened to the concept of self-efficacy, the belief that one can achieve desired outcomes through behaviors. In MS, the uncertainty of the disease course and the negative perception of the illness itself cause many people to feel hopeless and out of control. Patients' personal beliefs about their capacity to manage environmental demands will affect the course of action they choose to pursue. Personal beliefs will also affect how much effort they will expend, their length of perseverance, and how much anxiety or depression they will experience. A number of studies have documented that individuals with high self-efficacy are more likely to initiate and sustain a valuable activity (34).

Empowering Our Patients

The nurse working with patients and families can promote a feeling of self-efficacy utilizing the following strategies: (a) mastery over the environment, (b) vicarious experiences, (c) persuasive information, and (d) enhancement of physical and psychological states (36).

Mastery experiences are most effective in providing patients with a feeling of self-worth and accomplishment. A mastery experience involves the acquisition of tools for creating and implementing courses of action that may change life's circumstances.

Each indication of success helps to build a sense of personal efficacy or empowerment (34). For example, a person with MS who is successfully taught to manage his or her bowel or bladder dysfunction with dietary modifications, self-care activities such as catheterization, timed evacuations or voidings, and medications experiences mastery over the chaos wrought by this disease. This may, in turn, lead to future successful self-care activities related to the illness or other life situations.

Vicarious experiences or social modeling provide another way to create and strengthen patients' self-efficacy. Thus, reading about a successful activity, seeing it on television, or talking to another person in a similar circumstance can reinforce a person in a positive fashion. Others "in the same boat" can provide a standard against which to judge one's own capabilities. Models also can demonstrate skills and strategies for handling environmental demands (34).

Verbal persuasion by another is an important method of strengthening self-confidence in the ability to be successful. People who are persuaded that they are able to master an activity are more likely to persevere when problems arise (35).

Belief in oneself influences both a person's level of motivation and his or her tolerance for frustration or failure. Individuals who feel anxious should be taught to control stressors and mobilize coping strategies. People who learn to do so may view their environment with greater confidence, even though the same stressors may exist. Information giving is extremely important throughout the entire process of empowerment (35).

Patient and family empowerment is of profound importance to people with MS and is an important activity for the nurse in this field. Therapeutic actions to empower patients include the following (35):

- Facilitate goal setting that will allow for mastery experiences. These goals should be realistic, both short-term and long-term in nature, and should take all relevant factors into consideration. The establishment of multiple incremental goals is a motivational technique that encourages a person to strive toward a long-term goal.
- Provide experiences with other disabled people. Support groups provide opportunities for social modeling and for empathy by others who share similar feelings and experiences.
- Provide ongoing affirmation. "Cheerleading" is an important function of the nurse working with a patient who is facing a wide variety of challenges. It may consist of verbal "applause" or acknowledgment of both small and large accomplishments.
- Maximize physical and psychological functioning. Optimal physical and psychological functioning are essential components to the enhancement of self-worth. A fatigued and depressed person is more susceptible to a sense of diminished self-worth and is less apt to act on his or her own behalf.
- Provide motivation and encouragement that life has meaning. The nurse's professional ability to provide a patient with encouragement and a positive outlook is an essential art of caring. While presence and availability are crucial elements to encouragement, offering statements of faith can also be very beneficial.
- Provide personal belief in the ability to cope. Genuine concern about one's patient is an important feature of nursing care. A nonthreatening opening statement will invite your patient to share feelings and concerns. The nurse

TABLE 1-3
Empowering Ourselves and Those Affected by Multiple Sclerosis

• Be motivated	• Believe in yourself
• Find meaning in life experiences	• Develop effective coping strategies
• Communicate with others	• Find humor in your life
• Listen well and hear others	

can then elicit the patient's previous coping strategies and evaluate how effective they may be in the face of a chronic illness and/or disability.

Table 1-3 presents a tool that may be used by nurses to educate patients and families to empower them and to promote self-efficacy in their day-to-day dealings with MS.

Empowerment is essential for patients, families, and the healthcare provider in dealing with MS and its widespread implications. Self-efficacy, self-confidence, skills development, and effective communication are vital components and key features to promote successful coping with this perplexing and vexing chronic neurologic disease. The trick to empowerment is to learn and to teach others to focus not on "what was" but on "what can be."

Healthcare in Multiple Sclerosis

People with MS receive their care in a variety of settings (Table 1-4). Numerous professionals, functioning individually or as a team, may provide healthcare. Throughout their lifetimes, people with MS may interact with neurologists, nurses, rehabilitation professionals (physiatrists, physical or occupational therapists, or speech-language pathologists), counselors, educators, and/or members of community organizations such as MS organizations and their chapters.

Care Models in Multiple Sclerosis

Healthcare in MS has grown and evolved during the past 20 years as knowledge and interest in the disorder has increased as a result of advances in technology and the emergence of disease-modifying therapies.

Models of care in MS vary throughout the world. In the United States, MS patients receive primary care through specialist, rehabilitation, acute, home care, and long-term care settings. Insurance coverage ranges from Medicare, Medicaid, provate carriers, HMOs, and PPOs. In Canada, universal care is provided in a nationwide network of MS specialty programs, which are

TABLE 1-4
Models of Care in Multiple Sclerosis

Model	Clinical Features
Primary care provided by a family physician, internist, nurse practitioner, physician's assistant	Focuses on acute medical problems assesses for risk factors and treats them (medication education); care is episodic and not disease-specific; prevention and treatment of infections important in MS
*Specialty care**	
1. Neurologist	**1.** Diagnoses and treats MS
2. Urologist	**2.** Focuses on urologic dysfunction and sexual problems
3. Orthopedic	**3.** Treats musculoskeletal problems
4. Ophthalmologist	**4.** Assesses for visual disturbances, problems with the optic nerves, dysfunction of the ocular nerves
5. Physiatrist capabilities	**5.** Evaluates patients' physical and prescribes rehabilitation services, assistive devices, and mobility units
6. Psychiatrist	**6.** Assesses patients for emotional difficulties in dealing with MS, prescribes medications, and may give patients and families psychotherapy
7. Obstetrician/Gynecologist	**7.** Provides women with annual checkups, PAP smears, breast examinations; follows them throughout pregnancy and the postpartum period
Comprehensive care in MS	Collaborative practice, outreach into patients' homes, community, and workplace
A team of health professional who provide coordinated unduplicated services.	Addresses the spectrum of care needs in MS; physical, emotional, environmental, and/or vocational

*May be provided in one facility or many facilities.

supported by local primary care providers, home care programs, and long-term care settings (37).

Before the mid-1970s, care was fragmented and provided in many locations. Patients received the diagnosis and medical treatment by a neurologist, treatment of bladder problems by a urologist, physical therapy and other rehabilitation care in another facility, and, less frequently, mental health services and neuropsychological and vocational care somewhere else. The character of care at that time was "diagnose and adios." With the advent of MRI, that changed to "MRI and goodbye" (37).

There were few specialty MS programs or clinics in the United States and Canada until the early 1980s. There was little or no communication between healthcare providers and minimal continuity of services. Patients whose mobility or lack of transportation precluded access to care received no ongoing care except for emergencies. There were few MS specialty units, and care was fragmented, episodic, and related to crisis intervention instead of maintaining health. Treatment focused on symptomatic management, and disease modification was merely a dream. With the advent of MRI in the 1980s facilitating a more prompt diagnosis of MS, and the approval of disease-modifying therapies during the past decade, care patterns have changed not only in North America but also throughout the world. Initially, the emerging MS centers focused mainly on rehabilitation and its contribution to the maintenance of function and prevention of complications of the disease. Schapiro and Burks (38) were representative of a growing number of neurologists who recognized and embraced a comprehensive model of care in the United States while Paty and Murray similarly approached MS treatment in Canada. Since that time, comprehensive care in MS and in other chronic illnesses has been widely accepted as ideal.

Maintenance Rehabilitation Concept

Based on the increasing interest in MS rehabilitation, a concept defined as *maintenance rehabilitation* began to emerge. In a disease with no known cure, maintenance of function and productivity became a highly desirable outcome. This concept has gained credibility during the past two decades as more research began substantiating sustained benefit in patients who participated in rehabilitation services or a program of physical activity. The philosophic underpinnings of maintenance rehabilitation are to assist people with MS to take control of their lives no matter how severe the disease. The key is productivity and involvement for the disabled person and the reduction of social stigma and social isolation that usually result from alterations in physical or cognitive function. Schapiro has written that, whereas restorative rehabilitation focuses on crisis intervention and attainment of rehabilitation goals, maintenance rehabilitation "is prevention of a decrease in function whether directed toward a physical attribute or to emotional factors" (23).

Comprehensive Care in Multiple Sclerosis

Comprehensive care in MS is an organized system of healthcare designed to address the medical, social, vocational, emotional, and educational needs of patients and their families. This care is provided by a team of professionals, based in one facility, and tries to ensure that the direction and goals of treatment are consistent, logical, and progressive. The team approach facilitates coordination of services and continuity of care and avoids duplication and fragmentation for the patient and family. Comprehensive care embraces a philosophy of empowerment in which the patient takes an active role in planning and implementing healthcare and self-care activities and acts as consultant to the team. This active rather than passive role is fitting in light of the fact that MS, like all chronic illnesses, is expected to last a lifetime. Patients must learn to adapt and change in response to alterations in their physical functioning. This implies a total commitment to a clearly defined program of wellness that looks beyond impairments to what is possible for each person to achieve (38).

The Comprehensive Care Team

The comprehensive care team consists of a well-informed MS patient and his or her family or care partners; a neurologist and other physicians such as internists, physiatrists, urologists, gynecologists, orthopedists, ophthalmologists, psychiatrists; nurses, physicians' assistants, nurse practitioners, social workers, rehabilitation professionals, psychologists and neuropsychologists, recreational therapists, attorneys, and clergy. This interdisciplinary team evaluates each patient individually and develops a plan of care that reflects individual function with the patient's input. This plan of care reaches beyond center or clinic walls into homes, workplaces, and places of recreation to enable full and independent functioning and a full quality of life. This reflects the ever-changing healthcare, social, and emotional needs expressed by the patient (37).

The physician is responsible for the diagnosis and treatment of MS and the overall medical management of the patient's condition. He or she is obligated to communicate with the other team members, the patient, and the family about the plan of care (36).

The nurse, as an educator, informs patients and their families about the disease and their responsibility in treatment modalities such as bladder and bowel management, rehabilitation, and self-injection. Nursing care is individualized based on the patient's disease course, current complaints, and ability to handle new information. The nurse is a care provider performing hands-on procedures, a counselor assisting patients to get access to programs and services, and an advocate acting on behalf of patients and their families. In many instances, the nurse functions as an innovator who develops new programs such as support groups for newly diagnosed patients and families. This outreach function stretches beyond the confines of the clinic and centers and results in interactions with community agencies such as visiting nurse services, homemaker programs, MS society chapters, and other organizations that offer services for the disabled (38).

Physical therapists work with patients to improve strength and balance and gait, manage increased muscle tone, enhance coordination and ambulation using assistive devices and rehabilitative techniques, and promote compensation for sensory loss. In addition, they provide patients with the opportunity to utilize adaptive equipment for its suitability to their functional level (39).

Occupational therapists work with adaptive equipment and an exercise program mainly for the upper extremities. The therapist concentrates on the patient's activities of daily living and prior level of functioning, either vocationally or as a homemaker or student. The goals of occupational therapy are consistent with those of the team but are specific to maximal independence. Occupational therapists treat symptoms such as tremor and dystaxia with adaptive equipment and compensatory techniques to reduce dysfunction and promote independence wherever possible. Cognitive issues are also addressed in occupational therapy, especially as they affect the patient's ability to perform self-care activities or manage activities of daily living (39).

Speech-language pathologists focus on a variety of communication problems and potential medical problems such as swallowing difficulties and breathing problems. Symptoms such as dysarthria and poor voice projection can be addressed by a structured exercise program and regularly scheduled care. Communication patterns and thus the patient's self-esteem are improved. Dysphasia has recently been recognized as a potential problem in MS. Patients may be subject to silent aspiration, with resultant pulmonary complications. Therapy focuses on strengthening accessory muscles and instructing patients and their families to use alternate strategies for safe swallowing (39).

Counseling and supportive services may be provided by a social worker or a clinical psychologist and are designed to alleviate the stress of chronic illness. Counseling attempts to promote improved coping with the changes imposed by MS related to work, financial status, child care, relationships, and emotional responses by the patient and family. Attention to the psychological implications of the disease is as vital a component of comprehensive care as any other service or medication that may be prescribed (13).

In many comprehensive care centers, a neuropsychologist may be available to diagnose cognitive changes, a vocational counselor to assist patients in evaluating their employment status and vocational skills, and a recreation specialist to help develop new ways of relaxing and enjoying life despite MS (3). Social workers and case managers seek to identify and link patients with resources such as home care, transportation, and services to improve their quality of life.

Newly Emerging Patterns of Care

It has become increasingly evident that the nurse has a vital role to play in the ongoing care of and interaction with MS patients and their families.

The nurse has proven to be a vital partner in all settings, primarily in the comprehensive team model. This implies a total commitment to a clearly defined program of "wellness" that looks beyond impairments to each person's potential by the healthcare team and the patient (27). Nursing has found its way into new approaches to managing MS and other types of chronic illness.

One new approach to managing care in the United States is *case management*, which has been introduced as a cost-effective and efficient model for restructuring patient care delivery. Until the 1980s, healthcare in MS and other chronic diseases was fragmented, resulting in high costs and duplication of services. Since comprehensive care centers have proliferated throughout the world, their team approach has given new meaning to the case management model (40). A case manager or case coordinator coordinates patient care services provided by the interdisciplinary team and integrates healthcare services with community-based programs. This team player is usually a nurse (39) (see Chapter 10).

Clinical practice guidelines (CPGs) are the next logical step in providing dynamic care for this perplexing and ever-changing illness. CPGs—also called critical paths or pathways, collaborative plans of care, multidisciplinary action plans (MAPs), care paths, and anticipated recovery paths—are interdisciplinary plans of care that outline the optimal sequencing and timing of interventions for patients with a particular diagnosis, procedure, or symptom (39). They are designed to minimize delays while enhancing the utilization of resources and maximizing the quality of patient care. They include patient outcomes, time lines, collaboration, and comprehensive aspects of care (39,40)). In MS, the implementation of CPGs should reflect the dynamic nature of the illness in terms of the prognosis of the patient, the current state of health and function, and the resources available in the healthcare and residential communities. The development of CPGs in MS is a multinational and interdisciplinary approach to the management of the disease itself, its symptoms, and its long-term implications. It is an effort that was supported by numerous organizations involved in MS care and research and facilitated by the Paralyzed Veterans of America (PVA) in Washington, D.C. as the Multiple Sclerosis Council on Clinical Practice Guidelines. Guidelines for bladder management, fatigue, immunizations, and disease management are available for guidance and references (www.pva.org).

Summary

The nature of MS calls for dynamic and creative approaches to healthcare and requires a wide scope of skills and knowledge on the part of the healthcare team. The nurse has a vital role as a care provider, an educator of patients and their family members, an advocate, and a "linchpin" between team members, programs, and services. In the context of this positive approach, it is important to encourage patients to move out of a passive, "helpless" role into a proactive stance with regard to their disease. Using this strategy, there occurs a sense of empowerment in the context of the disease, a greater acceptance of a new "self," and an altered but reasonable view of the future. It is equally vital for an MS nurse to provide patients and families with accurate information in order to establish realistic expectations for proposed treatments, to educate patients in self-care and wellness, and to reestablish a sense of control over their bodies. A nurse's support, advice, education, and expertise can do much to advance MS from an incurable and uncontrollable disease to a set of manageable problems within the context of patients' lives. This positive approach can provide a firm foundation for coping with the challenges of MS over a lifetime.

REFERENCES

1.   Paty D, Ebers GC. *Multiple Sclerosis*. Philadelphia: FA Davis, 1998:135.
2.   Lublin FD, Reingold SC. Defining the clinical course of multiple sclerosis: Results of an international survey. *Neurology*. 1996;46:907–911.
3.   Coyle PK. Multiple sclerosis. In: Kaplan PK, ed. *Neurologic Disease in Women*. New York: Demos, 1998:251–264.
4.   Munschauer F. Presentation in Basel, Switzerland, September 1999.
5.   Lynch SG, Rose JW. Multiple sclerosis. In: Bone RC, ed. *Disease-a-Month*. St. Louis: Mosby-Year Book, 1996;42:3–55.
6.   Trapp BD, Peterson J, Ransahoff, et al. Axonal transection in the lesions of multiple sclerosis. *N Engl J Med*. 1998;338:287–285.
7.   Whetten-Goldstein K, Sloan FA, Goldstein LB, Kulas ED. A comprehensive assessment of the cost of multiple sclerosis in the United States. *Multiple Sclerosis*. 1998;4:419–425.
8.   Weinshenker BG, Bass B, Rice GPA, et al. The national history of multiple sclerosis: A geographically based study. 1. Clinical course and disability. *Brain*. 1989;112:133–146.
9.   Paty DW, Li DKB, UBC MS/MRI Study Group, IRNB Multiple Sclerosis Study Group. Interferon beta-1b is effective in relapsing-remitting multiple sclerosis. *Neurology*. 1993;43:662–667.
10. Poser CM, Paty DW, Scheinberg LC, et al. New diagnostic criteria for multiple sclerosis: Guidelines for research protocols. *Neurology*. 1983;13:227–231.
11. Polman CH, Reingold SC, Edan G, et al. Diagnostic criteria for multiple sclerosis: 2005 revisions to the "McDonald Critera." *Ann Neurol*. 2005 Dec; 58(6):840–6.
12. Thompson AJ, Kennard C, Swash M et al. Relative efficacy of intravenous methylprednisolone and ACTH in the treatment of acute relapse in MS. *Neurology*. 1989;39: 969–971.
13. Johnson KP, Brooks BR, Cohen JA, et al. Copolymer 1 reduces relapse rate and improves disability in relapsing-remitting multiple sclerosis: Results of a phase III multicenter, double-blind placebo controlled trial. *Neurology*. 1995;45:1268–1276.

14. Halper J, Holland NJ. An overview of multiple sclerosis: Implications for nursing practice. In: Halper J, Holland NJ, eds. *Comprehensive Nursing Care in Multiple Sclerosis.* New York: Demos, 2002.

15. LaRocca NG, Kalb RC. Psychosocial issues in multiple sclerosis. In: Halper J, Holland NJ, eds. *Comprehensive Nursing Care in Multiple Sclerosis.* New York: Demos, 2002.

16. Minden SL, Moees E. A psychiatric perspective in neurobehavioral aspects of multiple sclerosis. In: Rao SM, ed. *Neurobehavioral Aspects of Multiple Sclerosis.* New York: Oxford University Press, 1990:230–250.

17. Holland NJ. Patient and family education. In: Halper J, Holland, NJ, eds. *Comprehensive Nursing Care in Multiple Sclerosis.* New York: Demos, 2002.

18. Kalb RC. Psychosocial issues. In: Kalb RC, ed. *Multiple Sclerosis—The Questions You Have, The Answers You Need,* 3rd ed. New York: Demos, 2004.

19. Holland NJ, Kaplan SR. *Vocational Issues in Multiple Sclerosis: A Guide for Patients and Families,* 2nd ed. New York: Raven Press; 1987:229–237.

20. Halper J. Women's issues in multiple sclerosis. In: Halper J, Holland NJ, eds. *Comprehensive Nursing Care in Multiple Sclerosis.* New York: Demos, 2002.

21. Kalb RC, La Rocca NG. Sexuality and family planning. In: Halper J. Holland NJ, eds. *Comprehensive Nursing Care in Multiple Sclerosis.* New York: Demos, 2002.

22. LaRocca NG, Kalb RC. Psychosocial issues in multiple sclerosis. In: Halper J, Holland NJ, eds. *Comprehensive Nursing Care in Multiple Sclerosis.* New York: Demos, 2002.

23. The Multiple Sclerosis Nurse Specialists Consensus Committee. "Impact of Multiple Sclerosis on Quality of Life." *Multiple Sclerosis: Key Issues in Nursing Management,* 2nd ed. New York: Bioscience, 2004.

24. Petajan JH. Weakness. In: Burks JS, Johnson KP, eds. *Multiple Sclerosis: Diagnosis, Medical Management, and Rehabilitation.* New York: Demos; 2000:307–322.

25. Paty DW, Ebers GC. Clinical Features. In: Paty DW, Ebers GC, eds. *Multiple Sclerosis.* (CNS Series.) Philadelphia: FA Davis Co.; 1998:154, 159.

26. Schapiro RT, Schneider DM. Symptom management in multiple sclerosis. In: Halper J, Holland NJ, eds. *Comprehensive Nursing Care in Multiple Sclerosis.* New York: Demos, 2002.

27. Namey MA. Management of elimination dysfunction, In: Halper J, Holland NJ, eds. *Comprehensive Nursing Care in Multiple Sclerosis.* New York: Demos, 2002.

28. Weisel-Levison P, Halper J. Prevention of complications in the severely disabled patient. In: Halper J, Holland NJ, eds. *Comprehensive Nursing Care in Multiple Sclerosis.* New York: Demos, 2002.

29. Clark CC. *Wellness Nursing.* New York: Springer, 1986.

30. *The Random House Dictionary of the English Language.* New York: Random House, 1967:468.

31. Davidhizar R, Bechtel GA, Miller SW. Promoting self-efficacy in the chronically disabled client. *J Care Management.* 1998;4(2):44–62.

32. Ryan P. Facilitating behavior change in the chronically ill. In: Miller JF, ed. *Coping with Chronic Illness: Overcoming Powerlessness,* 2nd ed. Philadelphia: FA Davis, 1992.

33. Morgante LA. Hope: A unifying concept for nursing care in multiple sclerosis. In: Halper J, Holland NJ, eds. *Comprehensive Nursing Care in Multiple Sclerosis.* New York: Demos, 2002.

34. Jacobs M. Foster parent training: An opportunity for skills, enrichment and empowerment. *Child Welfare.* 1980;59(10):615–624.

35. Ford-Bilboe M. Family strengths, motivation, and resources as predictors of health promotion behavior in single-parent and two-parent families. *Res Nurs Health.* 1997; 20(30):205–217.

36. Davidhizar R, Bechtel GA, Miller SW. Promoting self-efficacy in the chronically disabled client. *J Care Manage.* 1998;4(2):44–62.

37. Schunk D. Self-efficacy and achievement behaviors. *Ed Psychol Rev.* 1989;1(2): 173–208.

38. Halper J, Burks JS. Care patterns in multiple sclerosis. *NeuroRehabilitation.* 1994 4(4): 67–75.

39. Cobble ND, Burks JS. The team approach to the management of multiple sclerosis. In: Maloney F, Burks JS, Ringel SR, eds. *Interdisciplinary Rehabilitation of Multiple Sclerosis and Neuromuscular Disorders.* Philadelphia: JB Lippincott; 1985:13.

40. Ignatavicius DD, Hausman KA. *Clinical Pathways for Collaborative Practice.* Philadelphia: WB Saunders, 1995.

41. Multiple Sclerosis Council for Clinical Practice Guidelines. Washington, DC: Paralyzed Veterans of America, 1998–2002.

CHAPTER 2

Therapeutic Advances in the Treatment of Progressive Forms of Multiple Sclerosis

Kathleen Costello

As described in Chapter 1, multiple sclerosis (MS) is a chronic disease of the central nervous system (CNS) that is usually diagnosed in the third or fourth decade of life, making it the most common neurologic disease of young adults. It has been generally accepted that MS is at least in part an immune-mediated disease. It is thought that peripherally activated T and B lymphocytes, as well as macrophages, which have the ability to recognize CNS proteins, enter the CNS and become reactivated. A cascade of immune system activity follows, including acute inflammation and the recruitment of additional immune active cells and substances that ultimately result in damage to myelin and the underlying nerve fibers (axons) (1).

Recently, it has been postulated that there may be additional pathologic mechanisms involved including immune and neural dysregulation within the CNS. For example, evidence suggests that activated microglia within the CNS may contribute to neurotoxicity and neurodegeneration (2). Glutamate is believed to be a neurotoxic substance, and Werner and coworkers have described alterations in glutamate that may contribute to myelin and axonal destruction (3).

New evidence from tissue samples suggest there may be more than one type of MS. Luchinetti and colleagues studied MS lesions and were able to identify four distinct patterns of damage. The damage was classified based upon inflammatory characteristics, remyelination present, the location of demyelination, and the status of oligodendrocytes. These were identified as patterns 1 through 4. The most common pattern (59.3% of sample) seen was pattern 2, which showed antibody-mediated inflammation greater than T-cell—mediated, preserved oligodendrocytes, perivenular demyelination and significant remyelination. In contrast, the next most common pattern, pattern 3 (25.9% of sample), showed concentric demyelination, less antibody-mediated inflammation, loss of oligodendrocytes, and poor remyelination (4). This important work provides information suggesting different mechanisms of damage, both inflammatory and degenerative. The now famous work by Trapp and colleagues (in 1998) demonstrated both early and late axonal damage in the brains of MS, indicating that a destructive and potentially degenerative process exists beyond the inflammatory response (5).

Some researchers believe that MS is a "dual-phase" disease (6), with one phase involving CNS damage from inflammation and one being a less understood degenerative process. It is the degenerative process that appears to be associated with clinical worsening and the more progressive characteristics of MS.

The clinical disease course in MS varies, and four courses were described by Lublin and Reingold (1995). These are defined as (7):

+ **Relapsing-remitting MS (RRMS),** characterized by periods of acute (new or returning) symptoms referable to the CNS, preceded by 30 days of stability and followed by some degree of recovery.
+ **Secondary progressive MS (SPMS),** characterized by gradual accumulation of disability following a period of relapsing-remitting disease that may or may not continue to be punctuated by relapses.
+ **Primary progressive MS (PPMS),** described as deterioration in function with increasing disability in the absence of relapses.
+ **Progressive-relapsing MS (PRMS),** characterized by progressive disease from onset, with the occurrence of a relapses after the progressive course has been established.

PPMS is felt by some to be a disease entity different from the relapsing forms of the disease. The presentation often includes more motor symptoms than seen at presentation in RRMS. The ratio of male to female patients with PPMS is approximately 1:1, versus the 1:3 seen in RRMS. Also, PPMS seems to develop at an older age, with onset often in the fifth decade (8). In addition, researchers have found that the CNS pathology demonstrated by magnetic resonance imaging (MRI) appears different in those with PPMS, with less cerebral lesions and less gadolinium enhancement (9).

Management of Multiple Sclerosis

Prior to 1993, the management of MS in the United States included treatment of acute relapses, symptomatic management, and limited off-label use of oral and intravenous immunosuppressive agents. The gold standard for the treatment of relapses was—and still is—high-dose glucocorticoids. Most ongoing treatment was symptomatic, aimed at symptoms such as fatigue, impaired mobility, and elimination dysfunction. In 1993, a new era in MS treatment began with the U.S. Food and Drug Administration's (FDA) approval of interferon beta-1b (Betaseron) for RRMS. For the first time an agent was able to alter the natural course of MS. This breakthrough was followed closely, in 1996, by the approvals of interferon beta-1a (Avonex) and glatiramer acetate for injection (Copaxone). In 2000, the FDA approved mitoxantrone (Novantrone) for the treatment of worsening MS. Mitoxantrone is an immunosuppressants agent and, although efficacious, carries greater risk than interferon or glatiramer acetate. In 2002, interferon beta-1a subcutaneous (Rebif) was approved in the United States for relapsing MS. Yet another treatment, natalizumab (Tysabri), was FDA approved for relapsing-remitting MS in late 2004. In early 2005, following the discovery of a potential link between natalizumab treatment and the development of progressive multifocal leukoencephalopathy, natalizumab was voluntarily withdrawn from the market. After much scrutiny, natalizumab was reapproved in mid-2006, with a black box warning and guidelines for patient selection and careful patient monitoring during treatment.

These disease modifying therapies changed the treatment paradigm of MS from reactive to highly proactive. These treatments target the errant immune system and act to reduce inflammation and relapses and, in some cases, delay progression of the disease. Glatiramer acetate, interferon beta-1b, and interferon beta-1a have all established long-term safety through ongoing open-label extensions of the Phase 3 trials. Due to the open-label design, lack of placebo control, retrospective analysis in some long-term trials, and the poor accounting of dropouts, long-term efficacy data are not as easily interpreted. Multiple sclerosis is now considered a treatable disease, and this fact has provided a sense of hope among providers and those living with the disease. In the years since the approvals of the disease-modifying treatments, many have seen the reduction of relapses and the delay of progression. However, the current therapies are only partially effective, and occasionally the response to treatment is suboptimal, thus leaving an unmet need in the treatment of MS.

The current treatments all have an effect on inflammation and are therefore most useful in relapsing MS. As stated earlier, it has been suggested that MS has both inflammatory and degenerative components. Progression in MS may be due in part to inflammation, but it is also due to the degenerative process that the current treatments are less able to address. Thus, treatment of SPMS and PPMS has been less successful, with modest benefit seen from mitoxantrone and interferon beta. Of the trials with interferon beta, only the European secondary-progressive MS trial demonstrated a positive effect on progression, as measured using the Expanded Disability Status Scale (EDSS) (10). The North American trial of interferon beta-1b, and trials of interferon beta- 1a (intramuscular, IM) and -1a (subcutaneous, SC) in SPMS failed to demonstrate efficacy in delaying or preventing progression (11–13). Both interferon beta-1a (IM) and 1a (SC) demonstrated a delay in disability in the relapsing MS populations (14,15). The success of interferon beta-1a in the RRMS populations and failure in SPMS may be an indication that there is more to MS than currently believed.

For those with more progressive disease, or those with relapsing disease for whom FDA-approved therapies have not been effective, other agents have been utilized. These treatments do not have an approved indication for MS, however they have immunosuppressive or immunomodulating activity that may favorably impact MS. Various small studies have indicated modest benefit in progressive forms of the disease. Although unapproved, it is not uncommon to see the use of off-label products either alone or in combination in clinical practice. Progression provokes fear in our patients and families. They often ask "When will I become progressive" or " Have I become progressive?" They see this as the road toward disability and, to a large extent, they are correct. Weinshenker and colleagues reported that 50% or more of relapsing patients will become secondary progressive within 10 years of disease onset. In 15 years, most will need some type of walking aid (16). In another longitudinal study by Confavreux and colleagues (16), the median time to EDSS 4.0 was 11.4 years and EDSS 6.0 was 23.1 years. At first glance, these endpoints seem to be long term, however, one must consider that a patient diagnosed at age 22 could have significant disability (EDSS of 4.0) by the age of 32 and an EDSS of 6.0 by the age of 45. Both of these endpoints occur within prime productivity years for family and career.

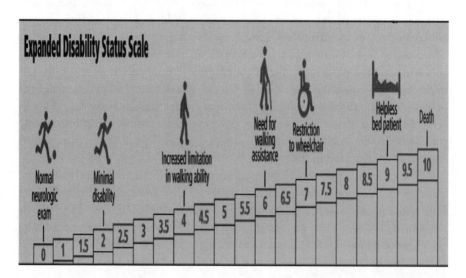

During the past 30 years, numerous agents have been utilized to treat progression or suboptimal response to FDA-approved therapies. Table 2-1 summarizes commonly prescribed unapproved agents. This is far from an exhaustive list, but it gives a sample of "off-label" agents.

The nurse involved in the care of patients with MS undoubtedly will encounter one or more of these unapproved agents. Patient care involving these agents must then be included in the nursing role.

Agents for Relapsing-Remitting and Secondary-Progressive Multiple Sclerosis

Azathioprine

Azathioprine (Imuran) is a derivative of mercaptopurine and is an antimetabolite immunosuppressant used to prevent rejection in renal homotransplantation and for the management of severe, refractory rheumatoid arthritis. It interferes with DNA and thus produces cell death of lymphocytes.

Azathioprine does not have an approved indication for the treatment of MS in the United States. However, it has been studied for use in MS since the 1970s, and multiple trials (17–23) have demonstrated modest benefit in treating the disease. Given orally, azathioprine may reduce relapses, but it does not seem to have a statistically significant effect on the progression of disability. Markovic-Plese and colleagues studied azathioprine in six MS patients for a median of 15 months and found a 69% reduction in gadolinium enhancement (24). In 2005, Puliken and colleagues reported treating 15 patients with breakthrough relapses on interferon beta-1b with the addition of azathioprine 3 mg/kg (dose escalated and titrated to tolerance) and demonstrated a 65% reduction in enhancing lesions, as demonstrated by serial MRI scans and compared with their precombination therapy level. EDSS remained unchanged. Of the 12 patients who completed the entire trial, nine had improvement in their Multiple Sclerosis Functional Competence (MSFC) score over the 6–month intervention phase of the study (25). Previously, in 2004, Massachesi and colleagues compared azathioprine at 3 mg/kg/d with interferon beta-1a 22 µg 3 times weekly in patients with relapsing MS and found similar reductions in gadolinium-enhancing lesions. Although the effect was anti-inflammatory, those who were worsening on monotherapy seemed to have some disease stabilization (26). Side effects of therapy include gastrointestinal (GI) upset, infection, hepatotoxicity, and anemia. Long-term therapy may increase the risk of developing certain malignancies.

TABLE 2-1
Sample of Immunomodulating and Immunosuppressant Agents

Trade Name	Generic Name	Indication/ Potential in MS	Side Effects	Selected Reference
Cytoxan	Cyclophosphamide	Antineoplastic agent used alone or in combination with other agents for the treatment of various types of cancer; disease stabilization	Leukopenia, thrombocytopenia, anemia, GI upset, alopecia	41, 42, 66
Imuran	Azathioprine	Adjunct for the prevention of rejection in renal homotransplantation; management of severe, active, rheumatoid arthritis; relapse reduction	Leukopenia, thrombocytopenia, nausea/vomiting, and pain, skin rashes, hepatotoxicity	21, 23
CellCept	Mycophenolate Mofetil	Prevention of transplant rejection	Bone marrow suppression	28
Leustatin	Cladribine	Antineoplastic agent for the treatment of active hairy cell leukemia; disease stabilization	Myelosuppression, with prolonged pancytopenia, mild to moderate infections, fever, nausea	44

Rheumatrex	Methotrexate	Antineoplastic agent used in variety of cancers, treatment of psoriasis, and rheumatoid arthritis; decreased rate of disease progression, particularly upper extremity function	Nausea, vomiting, diarrhea, anemia, leukopenia, thrombocytopenia, hepatoxicity, renal toxicity, lung disease	48
Sandoglobulin	Intravenous immunoglobulin	Treatment of immunodeficiencies; autoimmune neurologic diseases such as MG, CIDP; relapse reduction, delay of disease progression	During infusion: Facial flushing, chest tightness, chills, fever, dizziness, nausea, diaphoresis, and hypotension, anaphylaxis	30, 31, 67
Stem cell transplantation	Hematopoietic stem cell transplantation	Treatment of leukemia, lymphoma; induction of remission in progressive forms of MS	Infections, death, allergic reaction, transient worsening of neurologic symptoms	49, 68

Mycophenolate Mofetil

Mycophenolate mofetil (CellCept) inhibits inosine monophosphate dehydro-genase and blocks the proliferative ability of T and B cells. In addition, it has an effect on blocking antibody production in B cells. It may also have an effect on adhesion molecules (27). Several small studies have demonstrated favorable safety and tolerability and some indication of efficacy in terms of relapses and progression of dis-ability when used in combination with interferon or glatimer acetate. It is not FDA approved for the treatment of MS. Frohman and colleagues look ed retrospectively at 79 patients who had been given mycophenolate mofetil either alone or in com-bination with interferon beta or glatimer acetate. Sixty-one of these patients were considered to have SPMS. The authors found the drug to be relatively well tolerated and found that many patients reported stabilization or subjective improvement (28). Side effects include bone marrow suppression, anemia, and GI upset.

Intravenous Immunoglobulin

Intravenous immunoglobulin (IVIg) is approved for the treatment of primary immunodeficiencies and has been used in the treatment of a variety of autoimmune and immune-mediated diseases such as thrombocytopenia purpura, myasthenia gravis, and chronic inflammatory demyelinating polyneuropathy. It is not FDA approved for the treatment of MS. The mechanism of action is not well under-stood. In a recent study of 318 patients with active SPMS who were given IVIg every 4 weeks for 26 months, there was no benefit on time to EDSS progression, relapse rate, or MRI lesion load. There was, however, an effect on brain atrophy, with a significantly lower rate in the IVIg-treated patients (29).

Other previous studies by Fazekas and coworkers (30) and Achiron and colleagues (31) have shown that IVIg has a significant impact on relapse rate and some positive effect on disability. Side effects include thrombotic events, allergic reaction, headache, and aseptic meningitis syndrome. The most significant deterrents to widespread use of IVIG in MS are cost and limited supply when compared to evidence of modest benefit.

Intravenous Methylprednisolone

High-dose glucocorticoids, often intravenous or oral methylprednisolone, have been the mainstay of acute relapse intervention for the past 20 years. Although not FDA approved, many physicians report using intravenous methyl-prednisolone pulse therapy in some patients. High-dose glucocorticoids have anti-inflammatory properties and are believed to have a role in restoring integrity to the blood—brain barrier, as indicated by rapid reduction in gadolinium enhancement following administration (32).

In a study by Goodkin and colleagues, 108 patients with SPMS were given IVSM every other month for up to 2 years. The results demonstrated a modest effect in delaying sustained progression (33). In 2006, Bergh and colleagues reported a small study of nine RRMS patient given monthly IVSM and a brief oral taper. They showed a reduction in gadolinium enhancement and stable EDSS throughout the treatment period of 1 year (34).

Mitoxantrone

Mitoxantrone (Novantrone) is a potent immunosuppressant that reduces T cells, suppresses humoral immunity, and enhances suppressor function (35). It is the only FDA approved therapy for worsening and SPMS. It has additional indications for the treatment of pain related to hormone-refractory prostate cancer and the treatment of acute nonlymphocytic leukemia (36). It was found to be highly effective in the treatment of experimental allergic encephalomyelitis (EAE) (37). In a trial using intravenous mitoxantrone (20 mg per month) and intravenous methylprednisolone (1 gm per month) (38), patients in the mitoxantrone-methylprednisolone group showed fewer exacerbations, fewer enhancing lesions on MRI, and improvement in EDSS scores as compared with the methylprednisolone-alone group. In a trial conducted by Millefiorini and coworkers (39), mitoxantrone was compared with placebo in 51 patients with MS. Trial results demonstrated fewer exacerbations in the treatment group and less progression (by EDSS) in the 2—year evaluation. A Phase III trial of mitoxantrone in RR and SPMS demonstrated efficacy in MRI, relapses, and disability endpoints (40). Mitoxantrone is cardiotoxic, and the lifetime cumulative dose is 140 mg/m². Mitoxantrone increases the lifetime risk of certain cancers, such as acute myelogenous leukemia. It can cause bone marrow suppression, nausea, and fatigue. The FDA approved mitoxantrone in October 2000 for treatment of secondary progressive, progressive-relapsing, and worsening relapsing-remitting MS to reduce the frequency of relapses and reduce neurologic disability.

Cyclophosphamide

Cyclophosphamide is an alkylating immunosuppressant that acts to reduce cell proliferation. As an antineoplastic agent, it is used alone or in combination protocols in the treatment of various types of cancer. In addition, it has been investigated as potential treatment in MS based on its immunosuppressant activity. Clinical trial results have varied, and the agent is not approved for use in MS. Weiner and coworkers (41) found that pulse cyclophosphamide therapy following high-dose initiation with cyclophosphamide and adrenocorticotropic hormone slowed progression of the disease at the 24—month analysis. The results were modest and suggested that younger patients fared better in terms of disease stabilization. Goodkin and colleagues (42) found a trend toward disease stabilization in maintenance therapy using cyclophosphamide. Smith investigated the combination of cyclophosphamide 800 mg/m^2 and methylprednisolone in patients who continued to have disease activity on interferon beta. The outcomes of this small study were favorable, with less gadolinium enhancement and evidence of disease stabilization in the cyclophosphamide treated group (43). Cyclophosphamide was administered by intravenous infusion in these trials. It has numerous side effects, including leukopenia, neutropenia, nausea, vomiting, hemorrhagic cystitis, and alopecia.

Cladribine

Cladribine is a synthetic purine nucleoside analog and is indicated for the treatment of hairy cell leukemia. It is a synthetic agent administered intravenously or subcutaneously. It appears to work by accumulating in lymphocytes and damaging DNA repair and cell metabolism, which leads to cell apoptosis. It too, is not FDA approved for use in MS. In a Phase II double-blind, cross-over study Beutler and colleagues (44) found improved EDSS scores in the patients treated with cladribine compared with the same patients treated with placebo. The drug caused a reduction in CD4 cell counts, and this reduction was sustained beyond the treatment period. In another Phase II trial, subcutaneous cladribine was administered to 52 patients with RRMS. Patients received either cladribine or placebo for 5 consecutive days for six monthly courses. The study showed statistically significant outcomes in MRI, and the frequency and severity of clinical relapses (45). A Phase III trial of 159 patients given subcutaneous cladribine or placebo was reported in 2000 (46). The patients treated were characterized as SPMS and PPMS. The results did not show any effect on EDSS; however, this was felt to be in part by the stability of the placebo group. Further analysis did show some effect in the SPMS group. The MRI outcomes showed a reduction in enhancement and reduced T2 volumes.

Cladribine can produce thrombocytopenia, neutropenia, and anemia, and patients can be more susceptible to infections as a result of the prolonged leukopenia.

An oral form of cladribine is under study in a Phase III clinical trial being conducted in Europe and North America. This trial began recruitment in 2005. Both clinical and MRI endpoints are being studied.

Methotrexate

Methotrexate is an antimetabolite immunosuppressant that interferes with cell proliferation. Brody and colleagues 1 investigated methotrexate in inflammatory diseases and found that it interferes with the binding of interlocking 1, a cytokine that has been found to play an important roll in the inflammatory process and immune response (47).

Oral methotrexate in low doses is indicated for the treatment of rheumatoid arthritis and psoriasis, it is not however, approved for treatment of MS. A trial of 60 MS patients by Goodkin and coworkers (48) showed less progression in upper extremity functional loss in the treatment group. Treatment consisted of oral methotrexate, 7.5 mg given weekly for 2 years. Methotrexate can cause nausea, diarrhea, alopecia, pulmonary fibrosis, anemia, and liver toxicity.

Stem Cell Transplantation

Stem cell transplantation is aggressive, experimental treatment for patients with certain types of cancers such as breast carcinoma, leukemia, and lymphoma. In MS, it is thought that complete immunosuppression followed by stem cell transplantation may allow for proliferation of less autoreactive cells and therefore less MS activity (19). A small study of three patients by Burt and coworkers (49) demonstrated stabilization and some improvement in neurologic function. The procedure used in this study included bone marrow collection from the iliac crest followed by patient conditioning with cyclophosphamide, total body irradiation, and intravenous methylprednisolone. Conditioning was followed by autologous stem cell transplantation. In 2001, Mancardi reported autologous stem cell transplantation in 10 patients with SPMS. Patients were followed for 15 months, and did show clinical stabilization and a reduction in gadolinium enhancement, particularly following the cyclophosphamide pretransplant treatment. Brain atrophy did continue however (50). In another study of 60 SPMS patients treated with autologous stem cell transplantation, retrospective analysis showed that 66% had stability at 3 years (51). Although these results are encouraging, it is important to note that mortality from this procedure is approximately 5% to 10%, and the cost of the procedure is very high.

Agents for Primary-Progressive Multiple Sclerosis

Although no therapy has been found through clinical trials to be effective in PPMS, numerous trials have been conducted looking for effect on disability with the use of interferon beta-1a IM, interferon beta-1a SC, interferon beta-1b SC, and daily subcutaneous glatimer acetate (52,53). Unfortunately, no effect was demonstrated on EDSS. A large Phase III trial of glatimer acetate in 943 primary progressive patients was stopped early, because there was no statistically significant result possible if the study were carried to completion (54). The primary endpoint of this trial was EDSS.

Zephir and colleagues looked retrospectively at 490 patients treated with cyclophosphamide and methylprednisolone. Of the entire group, 128 had PPMS and 73.9% showed clinical stabilization over 1 year. The results must be interpreted cautiously because the study design was retrospective and open-label. Still, it does provide some indication to efficacy in PPMS (55).

Riluzole is an agent that has some effect on prolonging survival in amyotrophic lateral sclerosis (ALS). It has an effect on glutamate activity, which has a role in neurotoxicity. A small 16–patient study of riluzole given orally demonstrated cord stabilization by MRI measures in the second year (56). This agent may have neuroprotective properties, and could move MS research into a new direction.

Autologous stem cell transplant in 85 progressive MS patients—22 with PPMS—showed 66% with clinical stabilization at 3 years. Unfortunately, two deaths occurred in the PPMS treated groups, clearly a major limitation to the widespread use of this treatment (57).

A large Phase III trial of rituximab in PPMS is currently under way. Rituximab is an anti-CD20 monoclonal antibody, thus a B-cell inhibitor, and it is thought to be potentially beneficial in PPMS.

Summary of Therapies

Various immunosuppressant agents have been attempted in the treatment of MS with variable results. Although most results are modest, they are suggestive of benefit. Administration protocols differ, and side effects can be profound. There is tremendous interest in the MS research community regarding immuno-suppression either alone or in combination with other agents. Numerous trials are ongoing and are looking at the safety of combinations and the efficacy in terms of relapse control, effect on progression, and effect on MRI parameters. The MS nurse specialist must be familiar with these therapies to offer the best possible care for patients.

Education in Progressive MS

"Patient education is the deliberative process of creating behavioral and cognitive change in patients" (58). However, this is far from a one-sided process. It is accomplished with the combination of a prepared educator and a motivated, ready learner. Education of the patient with MS and those significant to the patient is critical. Bandura's social learning theory speaks to the importance of the individual and the social process of learning. This theory, which is based on behaviorist and cognitive theory, views learning as occurring in four steps: attentional, retentional, reproductive, and motivational (59,60). In this theory, the educator must pay attention to the social environment, the behavior to be performed, and the individual learner (61). This theory has logical application to MS patient education.

Holland (62) describes the educational goals in MS as:

+ Understanding the diagnosis and successfully coping with its potential impact on one's life
+ Planning regarding critical areas such as relationships, parenting, employment, and lifestyle
+ Preventing potentially disabling outcomes, with specific goals related to new symptoms

As with other chronic illnesses, the patient must learn to adapt to changes over time. These changes involve self, family, employment, and community roles. The medical team must be collaborators with the patient, not the dictator in the efforts to manage the disease and its implications. For optimal wellness, the individual with the diagnosis must be in charge. Knowledge can promote wellness and minimize the negative effects of the disease (63). The healthcare team functions as an assistant to the patient's independence.

Dissemination of information is a critical element in MS care. The nurse caring for those with MS must provide information to the patient, the family, other healthcare providers, and herself. Education begins during the diagnostic process and continues indefinitely. The newly diagnosed person and family require accurate information regarding the diagnostic process, the disease, and the currently approved therapies. They must be steered toward useful literature and Internet sources. The nurse should encourage questions and provide for additional education sessions. Invariably, the overwhelming nature of the diagnosis will preclude absorption of all information, and the nurse should expect the need for follow-up sessions. Referral to the National Multiple Sclerosis Society, and other patient advocacy groups, for ongoing education and resources provides useful and credible sources of information and support. Families often have educational needs that are different from those of the patient. Although families require factual information, they also need help understanding the disease. Many symptoms of MS are "invisible" to anyone other than the patient. The nurse must make an effort to help the family understand the patient's reality, not to focus only on what can be seen externally. Family members must learn how they can be supportive to the patient, both physically and emotionally.

The MS nurse specialist must be able to educate other nurses involved in the care of those with the disease, including nursing students, home care nurses, hospital-based nurses, and case managers. These nurses need up-to-date information regarding new findings about the disease process and new agents for disease modification and symptom management.

Progressive MS produces fear and anxiety for patients and families. The nursing care needs in progressive MS can be complex. It is important to maintain a positive therapeutic relationship between the nurse and patient. Physical and cognitive decline are common in progressive MS, and the nurse, physician, patients, and family must work together as care needs and therapeutic interventions change. The nurse will encounter both approved and unapproved agents during the care of MS patients. Experimentation with unapproved agents begins because of suboptimal response to approved therapies. The nurse must be aware of the approved indication for the agent and why it is thought to work in MS. Patients must know the realistic expectations of the unapproved agent. Young and Brooks (64) found that patients who were given written information had greater retention of the information than those given verbal communication alone. Thus, literature regarding the agent, particularly its use in MS, will be useful to the patient and family.

Most of the unapproved agents for MS disease management are immunosuppressants, which have a myriad of side effects and risks. The patient and family must have a clear understanding of these adverse effects and risks. Many institutions require a consent form with the use of immunosuppressants, further emphasizing the need for education.

Finally, the patient must be aware of the need for close follow-up after the administration of unapproved agents. Among other side effects, immunosuppressants can cause bone marrow suppression, therefore frequent laboratory tests are necessary. In addition, the neurologic effect of the treatment must be monitored.

Advocacy in Progressive MS

The concept of the nurse as a patient advocate is far from new. Nurses have been working for the rights of patients as long as the profession has been in existence. The complex nature of a long-term, chronic illness is the perfect territory for advocacy. Price (65) wrote that the nurse is uniquely qualified to be an advocate for patients, and in MS that role includes:

+ Championing individual patient rights
+ Supporting changes in institutional or agency rules and regulations
+ Fostering health policy reforms
+ Promoting the rights of people with disabilities

Through successful efforts of the nurse as an advocate, the patient gains independence and becomes empowered.

The nurse advocate acts on the ethical principles of nonmalfeasance, beneficence, autonomy, and confidentiality. *Nonmalfeasance* is to prevent harm to the patient and is the overriding principle of the nursing profession. Nurses must be alert to any interventions that could be harmful. *Beneficence*, or to do good, is the attempt to help the patient to a higher level of function. *Autonomy* is the right of the patient to be treated as an individual and to have the right to choose treatment or alternatives to treatment. *Confidentiality* requires that any information pertaining to the patient be protected.

Advocacy has several implications when unapproved therapies are considered. The ethical principles described previously must guide the actions of the nurse. Of the utmost importance is nonmalfeasance, or to do no harm. The nurse must be aware of the risks of unapproved therapies and ensure that the patient clearly understands them. The nurse should question therapies when the risk may outweigh the potential benefit. When risk appears to outweigh benefit, the nurse should consult the hospital ethics committee for guidance.

Beneficence dictates that the nurse should make the patient aware of therapies or treatments that have potential benefit. The patient's right to autonomy requires the nurse to ensure the patient has correct information and to support the decision making of the patient. Many third-party payers in the United States are reluctant to provide coverage for experimental therapies. They must weigh the risks and benefits for their interests as well as those of the patient. When evidence exists that supports safe, beneficial use of an unapproved agent, the nurse must act on behalf of the patient and appeal to the insurer to provide coverage. This requires knowledge of the therapies and the literature that supports their use in MS. This advocacy for access to treatment can extend to the legislative process, through which nurses can lobby for patients to have access to useful unapproved agents.

Approved and unapproved pharmaceutical interventions are an important part of the care plan for progressive MS. However, equally important are the interventions of other members of the comprehensive care team such as physical therapists, occupational therapists, social workers, and medical specialists such as urologists. The nurse advocate must keep patients and families well informed and connected to the care team, whether it exists under one roof or extends into the community.

Summary

Breakthroughs came in rapid succession during the 1990s, yet the cure for MS remains elusive. Until our approved interventions can eliminate the devastating outcomes of the disease, unapproved agents will continue to be a part of the management of MS.

Multiple sclerosis is a complex disease with physical, emotional, and social ramifications for both patients and families. Through education, support, and advocacy, the nurse can empower patients and families adjust to illness, understand therapies, and maintain a high quality of life.

REFERENCES

1. Raine CS. The Dale E. McFarlin Memorial Lecture: The immunology of the multiple sclerosis lesion. *Ann Neurol.* 1994;36(Suppl):S61–S72.

2. Imitola J, Chitnis T, Khoury SJ. Insights into the molecular pathogenesis of progression in multiple sclerosis: Potential implications for future therapies. *Arch Neurol.* 2006;63:25–33.

3. Werner P, Pitt D, Raine CS. Multiple sclerosis: Altered glutamate homeostasis in lesions correlates with oligodendrocyte and axonal damage. *Ann Neurol.* 2001;50:169–180.

4. Lucchinetti C, Brück W, Parisi J, et al. Heterogeneity of multiple sclerosis lesions: implications for the pathogenesis of demyelination. *Ann Neurol.* 2000;47:707–717.

5. Trapp BD, Peterson J, Ransohoff RM, et al. Axonal transection in the lesions of multiple sclerosis. *N Engl J Med.* 1998;338:278–285.

6. Dhib-Jalbut S. Personal communication. 2006.

7. Lublin RD, Reingold SC. Defining the clinical course of multiple sclerosis: Results of an international survey. *Neurology.* 1996;46:907–911.

8. Thompson AJ, Polman CH, Miller DH, et al. Primary progressive multiple sclerosis. *Brain.* 1997;120:1085–1096.

9. Revesz T, Kidd D, Thompson AJ, et al. A comparison of the pathology of primary and secondary progressive multiple sclerosis. *Brain.* 1994;117:759–765.

10. Kappos L, Polman C, Pozzilli C, et al. European Study Group in Interferon beta-1b in Secondary-Progressive MS. Final analysis of the European multicenter trial on IFNbeta-1b in secondary-progressive MS. *Neurology.* 2001;57(11):1969–1975.

11. Panitch H, Miller A, Paty D, et al. North American Study Group on Interferon beta-1b in Secondary Progressive MS. Interferon beta-1b in secondary progressive MS: Results from a 3-year controlled study. *Neurology.* 2004;63(10):1788–1795.

12. Secondary Progressive Efficacy Clinical Trial of Recombinant Interferon beta-1a in MS (SPECTRIMS) Study Group. Randomized controlled trial of interferon beta-1a in secondary progressive MS: Clinical results. *Neurology.* 2001;56:1496–1504.

13. Cohen JA, Cutter GR, Fischer JS, et al. and IMPACT investigators. Benefit of interferon beta-1a on MSFC progression in secondary progressive MS. *Neurology.* 2002;59:679–687.

14. Jacobs LD, Cookfair DL, Rudick RA, et al. and the Multiple Sclerosis Collaborative Research Group (MSCRG). Intramuscular interferon beta-1a for disease progression in relapsing multiple sclerosis. *Ann Neurol.* 1996;39(3):285–294.

15. PRISMS (Prevention of Relapses and Disability by interferon beta-1a Subcutaneously in Multiple Sclerosis) Study Group. Randomized double-blind placebo-controlled study of interferon beta-1a in relapsing-remitting multiple sclerosis. *Lancet.* 1998;352(9139):1498–1504.

16. Weinshenker B, Bass B, Rice G, et al. The natural history of multiple sclerosis: A geographically based study. *Brain.* 1989;112:133–146.

17. Confavreux C, Vukusic S, Moreau T, Adeleine P. Relapses and progression of disability in multiple sclerosis. *N Engl J Med.* 2000;343:1430–1438.

18. Silberberg DH, et al. Multiple sclerosis unaffected by azathioprine in pilot study. *Arch Neurol.* 1973;3:210–212.

19. Swinburn WR, Liversedge LA. Long-term treatment of multiple sclerosis with azathioprine. *J Neurol Neurosurg Psychiatry.* 1973;36:124–126.

20. Zeeburg IE, Heltberg A, Fog T. Follow-up evaluation after at least two years' treatment with azathioprine in a double-blind trial. *Eur Neurol.* 1985; 24:435–436.

21. British and Dutch Multiple Sclerosis Azathioprine Trial Group. Double masked trial of azathioprine efficacy in multiple sclerosis: Preliminary results. *Ital J Neurol Sci.* 1988;9:53–57.

22. Ellison GW, Myers LW, Mickey MR, et al. A placebo-controlled, randomized, double masked, variable dosage, clinical trial of azathioprine with and without methylprednisolone in multiple sclerosis. *Neurology.* 1989;39:1018–1026.

23. Goodkin DE, Bailly RC, Teetzen ML, et al. The efficacy of azathioprine in relapsing remitting multiple sclerosis. *Neurology.* 1991;41:20–25.

24. Markovic-Plese S, Bielekova B, Kadom N, et al. The effects of azathioprine n MS patients refractory to interferon beta-1b. *Neurology.* 2003;60:1849–1851.

25. Pulicken M, Bash CN, Costello K, et al. Optimization of the safety and efficacy of interferon beta 1b and azathioprine combination therapy in multiple sclerosis. *Multiple Sclerosis.* 2005;11(2):169–174.

26. Massachesi L, Barilaro A, Repice A, et al. Comparison of azathioprine and interferon beta1a efficacy on prevention of new brain lesions in relapsing remitting multiple sclerosis. *Program and abstracts of the 56th Annual Meeting of the American Academy of Neurology.* April 24–May 1, 2004; San Francisco, California. Abstract PO4.036.

27. Product monograph. Mycophenolate mofetil. Roche Laboratories.

28. Frohman EM, Brannon K, Racke MK, Hawker K. Mycophenolate mofetil in multiple sclerosis. *Clin Neuropharmacol.* 2004;27(2):80–83.

29. Hommes OR, Sorensen PS, Fazekas F, et al. Intravenous immunoglobulin in secondary progressive multiple sclerosis: Randomised placebo-controlled trial. *Lancet.* 2004;364: 1149–1156.

30. Fazekas F, Deisenhammer F, Strasser-Fuchs S, et al., for the Austrian Immunoglobulin in Multiple Sclerosis Study Group. Intravenous immunoglobulin therapy in relapsing-remitting multiple sclerosis treatment in MS. Effects on relapses. *Neurology.* 1998;50: 398–402. *Lancet.* 1977;349:589–593.

31. Achiron A, Gabby U, Gilad R, et al. Intravenous immunoglobulin treatment in MS. Effects on relapses. *Neurology.* 1998;50:398–402.

32. Barkhof F, Hommes OR, Scheltens P, Valk J. Quantitative MRI changes in gadolinium-DTPA enhancement after high-dose intravenous methylprednisolone in multiple sclerosis. *Neurology.* 1991;41:1219–1222.

33. Goodkin DE, Kinkel RP, Weinstock-Guttman B, et al. A phase II study of IV methylprednisolone in secondary-progressive multiple sclerosis. *Neurology.* 1998;51:239–245.

34. Then Bergh, Kumpfel T, Schumann E, et al. Monthly intravenous methylprednisolone in relapsing remitting multiple sclerosis-reduction of enhancing lesions, T2 lesion volume and plasma prolactin concentrations. *BMC Neurology.* 2006;6(19):1471–2377.

35. Fidler JM, Quinn De Joy S, Gibbonson JJ. Selective immunomodulation by the antineoplastic agent mitoxantrone. *J Immunol.* 1986;137:727–732.

36. Novantrone, mitoxantrone for injection concentrate. Full prescribing information. *Physician's Desk Reference*, 53rd, ed., Thomson PDR, Montvale, NJ, 2007.

37. Ridge SC, Sloboda AE, Reynolds RA, et al. Suppression of experimental allergic encephalomyelitis by mitoxantrone. *Clin Immunol Immunopathol*. 1985;35:35–42.

38. Edan G, Miller D, Clanet M, et al. Therapeutic effect of mitoxantrone combined with methylprednisolone in multiple sclerosis: A randomized multicenter study of active disease using MRI and clinical criteria. *J Neurol Neurosurg Psychiatry*. 1997;62:112–118.

39. Millifiorini E, et al. Randomized, placebo-controlled trial of mitoxantrone in relapsing-remitting MS. 24–month clinical and MRI outcome. *J Neurol*. 1997;244:153–159.

40. Hartung HP, Gonsette R, Konig N. Mitoxantrone in progressive multiple sclerosis: A placebo-controlled, double blind, randomized, multicenter trial. *Lancet*. 2002;360:2018–2025.

41. Weiner HL, Mackin glatimer acetate, Orav EJ, et al., and the Northeast Cooperative Multiple Sclerosis Treatment Group. Intermittent cyclophosphamide pulse therapy in progressive multiple sclerosis: Final report of the northeast cooperative multiple sclerosis treatment group. *Neurology*. 1993;43:910–918.

42. Goodkin DE, Plencner S, Palmer-Saxerud J, et al. Cyclophosphamide in chronic-progressive multiple sclerosis, maintenance vs. nonmaintenance therapy. *Arch Neurol*. 1987;44:823–827.

43. Smith D. Preliminary analysis of a trial of pulse cyclophosphamide in interferon β-resistant active MS. *J Neurolog Sci*. 2004;223(1):73–79.

44. Beutler E, et al. The treatment of chronic progressive multiple sclerosis with cladribine. *Proc Natl Acad Sci USA*. 1996;93:1716–1720.

45. Romine JS, Sipe JC, Koziol JA, et al. A double-blind, placebo controlled, randomized trial of cladribine in relapsing-remitting multiple sclerosis. *Proc Assoc Am Physicians*. 1999;111:35–44.

46. Rice GP, Filippe M, Comi G. Cladribine and progressive MS: Clinical and MRI outcomes of a multicenter controlled trial. Cladribine MRI Study Group. *Neurology*. 2000;54:1145–1155.

47. Brody M, Bohm I, Bauer R. Mechanism of action of methotrexate: Experimental evidence that methotrexate blocks the binding of interleukin 1 beat to the interleukin 1 receptor on target cells. *Eur J Chem Clin Biochem*. 1993;31(10):667–674.

48. Goodkin DE, Rudick R, VanderBrug-Medendorp S, et al. Low-dose (7.5 mg) oral methotrexate reduces the rate of progression in chronic progressive multiple sclerosis. *Ann Neurol*. 1995;37:30–40.

49. Burt RK, Traynor AE, Cohen B. T cell depleted autologous hematopoietic stem cell transplantation for multiple sclerosis. Report on the first three patients. *Bone Marrow Transplant*. 1998;21:537–541.

50. Mancardi Gl, Saccardi R, Filippi M, et al. Italian GITMO_NEURO Intergroup on Autologous Stem Cell Transplantation for Multiple Sclerosis. Autologous hematopoietic stem cell transplantation suppresses Gd-enhanced MRI activity in MS. *Neurology*. 2001;57:62–68.

51. Fassas A, Passwer JR, Anagnostopoulos A, et al., and the Autoimmune disease Working Party of the European Group for Blood and Marrow Transplantation. Hematopoietic stem cell transplantation for multiple sclerosis: A retrospective multicenter study. *J Neurol*. 2002;249:1088–1097.

52. Leary SM, Miller DH, Stevenson VL. Interferon beta-1a in primary progressive MS. An exploratory, randomized, controlled trial. *Neurology.* 2003;60:44–51.

53. Montalban X. Overview of European pilot study of interferon beta-1b in primary progressive multiple sclerosis. *Multiple Sclerosis.* 2004;S1:62.

54. Wolinsky JS. The diagnosis of primary progressive multiple sclerosis. *J Neurolog Sci.* 2003;206(2):145–152.

55. Zephir H, deSeze J, Huhamel A. Treatment of progressive forms of multiple sclerosis by cyclophosphamide: A cohort study of 490 patients. *J Neurolog Sci.* 2004;218:73–77.

56. Kalkers NF, Barkhof F, Bergers E. The effect of the neuroprotective agent riluzole on MRI parameters in primary progressive multiple sclerosis: A pilot study. *Multiple Sclerosis.* 2002;8:532–533.

57. Fassas A, Passweg JR, Anagnostopoulos A. Hematopoietic stem cell transplantation for multiple sclerosis: A retrospective multicenter study. *J Neurol.* 2002;249:1088–1097.

CHAPTER 3

Optimal Primary Care Management for People with Multiple Sclerosis

June Halper

Wellness and the maintenance of general health are often overlooked by people who are confronted with the day-to-day challenges of chronic illness and disability. The diagnosis and treatment of multiple sclerosis (MS) is traditionally provided in a neurologic setting. Thereafter, healthcare tends to be focused on the disease, with primary care needs taking a back seat. This appears to stem both from the patient's increasing immobility, which may preclude access to healthcare facilities, and from knowledge deficits regarding primary care needs. Multiple sclerosis is a complex condition that is particularly sensitive to problems in the patient's health state (1). Therefore, primary care needs should be met in a timely and effective manner. The nurse, who is often the key member of the healthcare team, is in an excellent position to ensure that this occurs.

Maintaining a Balanced Health State

Annual physical examinations are as important for those with MS as for the general population. It is important that patients be given full physical assessments and age- and gender-appropriate diagnostic tests (Table 3-1).

TABLE 3-1
Guidelines for Adult Screening

Procedure	Women <50	50–64	>65	Men <50	50–60	>65
Screening						
Blood pressure	Annually	Annually	Annually	Annually	Annually	Annually
Cholesterol	Once	Every 5 yrs	Every 5 yrs	Once	Every 5 yrs	Every 5 yrs
Fecal blood	—	Annually	Annually	—	Annually	Annually
Sigmoidoscopy	—	Every 5–10 yrs	Every 5–10 yrs	—	Every 5–10 yrs	Every 5–10 yrs
CBE	Annually after 40	Annually	Annually			
Mammography	Every 1–2 yrs	Every 1–2 yrs	Every 1–2 yrs to 75			
Pap	Every 3 yrs if sexually active	Every 3 yrs if sexually active	Every 3 yrs to 75			
Vision	Annually	Annually	Annually	Annually	Annually	Annually
Hearing	Every 5 yrs	Every 5 yrs	Every 5 yrs	Every 5 yrs	Every 5 yrs	Every 5 yrs
PPD	Patient at risk	Patient at risk	Patient at risk			
Immunizations						
Td	Every 10 yrs	Every 10 yrs	Every 10 yrs	Every 10 yrs	Every 10 yrs	Every 10 yrs
Influenza*	Patient at risk (annually)	Patient at risk (annually)	Annually	Annually	Annually	Annually
Pneumococcal*	Patient at risk (once)	Patient at risk (once)	Once	Patient at risk (once)	Patient at risk (once)	Once

	Annual Counseling					
Smoking	+	+	+	+	+	+
Exercise	+	+	+	+	+	+
Diet						
Calcium Intake	+		+			+
Fat			+			+
Sex Education	+	+	+	+	+	+
Depression			+		+	+
Injury Prevention			+		+	+
Alcohol/Driving	+	+	+	+	+	+

*See complete recommendations, pp. 90–91.

CBE, clinical breast examination; PPD, purified protein derivative; Td, tetanus/diphtheria.

Used with permission from Hoole AJ, Pickard CG, Ouimette R, Lohr JA, Powell, WI. *Patient Care Guidelines for Nurse Practitioners*, 5th ed. Philadelphia: Lippincott Williams & Wilkins, 1999:82.

Increasing evidence points to the importance of maintaining an appropriate immunization schedule well into adulthood, along with appropriate seasonal and risk-reducing vaccines (influenza and Pneumovax) (2). A full health history will yield information about specific risk factors in the patient's genetic background as well as in his or her lifestyle, and these may be reduced with appropriate education and information. Certainly, MS should not preclude self-care activities to promote adequate and balanced nutrition, activity and exercise, and stress management. Women should be encouraged to perform breast self-examinations on a monthly basis; those with limited hand dexterity should be encouraged to enlist the help of their partner or significant other to perform this important evaluation. Men, particularly those in their twenties and thirties, should be taught to do testicular self-examinations; similarly, assistance and education should be provided to them if hand function is a problem (2).

Hormonally Mediated Events

Pregnancy

Pregnancy appears to have a protective effect on MS, whereas the postpartum period is one of high risk for exacerbations. This phenomenon is poorly understood but is well documented in the literature. Therefore, it is particularly important for MS patients and their families to consider the following during the intrapartum period:

- The patient's physical capabilities before conception
- Available family and other support systems in helping to care for the new baby
- Considerations regarding breast-feeding, bottle-feeding, and fatigue
- The patient's and family's living situation and economic resources

Pre- and postnatal counseling and support are particularly important to guarantee adequate rest, avoidance of infections, and management of the stress incumbent on first-time parents. Education of the patient and family, collaboration with obstetricians regarding the aforementioned concerns, and careful planning are essential in assisting young women and men to successfully achieve parenthood when MS affects the family (3).

Menstrual Cycle

Many women report a premenstrual increase in their symptoms, or what they describe as an *exacerbation*, and a relief of these symptoms once menstrual bleeding begins. It is important that the primary care physician and/or the nurse identify the patient's premorbid menstrual cycle (premenstrual syndrome, cramping, bloating, etc.), current medications (corticosteroids, immunomodu-lating medications, antispasticity agents), activity level, and diet. Collaboration with a gynecologist and neurologist who understand MS and its gynecologic implications may be extremely helpful in assisting the patient to manage this particularly difficult area. Strategies that may be helpful in symptom reduction might include dietary changes, moderate exercise, oral contraception, or medica-tions such as nonsteroidal anti-inflammatory drugs (NSAIDs).

Menopause

The effects of menopause on MS is under-researched. In an illness that can affect cognition, there is little evidence other than anecdotal about changes that may occur with diminished hormonal production and normal aging processes. Issues such as genital changes (vaginal dryness, diminished libido), an increased risk of osteoporosis, a higher incidence of cardiovascular disease, and other chronic conditions are not well understood. Aging women and men with MS require indi-vidualized assessments and interventions to prevent other chronic conditions from negatively impacting their quality of life. Special healthcare services for the aging disabled are strongly recommended to provide this care. Education and support are equally as important in the aging MS population as in younger MS populations (3).

Recognizing and Preventing Pseudoexacerbations

Numerous sources have suggested that infections and increased body temperature are significant precipitating events for relapses. Recommendations should include:

- Avoid increasing core body temperature (fever).
- Maintain body coolness with cooling devices, cool drinks, and cool showers if the ambient temperature is high.
- Cool down frequently while exercising, and exercise in a cool environment.
- Swimming is a healthful and appropriate exercise in MS.

The physician should reassure patients that no permanent damage is done to the nervous system by exposure to heat, but that the patient may be at risk of falls and/or injury because of increased symptoms and perhaps weakness.

It is well documented that exacerbations of MS are frequently preceded by viral infections and/or upper respiratory tract infections. A recent study has shown no evidence of neurologic deterioration after influenza vaccination, so it is recommended that susceptible individuals, particularly those with disabling MS, be advised to be vaccinated against influenza at the appropriate season. People with significant disease may be well advised to be vaccinated against pneumonia as well. Amantadine may provide an alternative for influenza prophylaxis, and also may reduce symptoms of fatigue (4).

It is extremely important to recognize and treat infections promptly. Urinary tract infections (UTIs) are probably the most common infection encountered with MS, although one might find dental abscesses, skin infections, or tonsillitis likely culprits in causing pseudoexacerbations. Once fever is reduced and the infection is under control, MS symptoms that may have flared and frightened the patient will remit to baseline.

The healthcare provider should promptly ascertain the cause of elevated body temperature, particularly in this era of immunomodulating therapies. Interferons, particularly during the early stages of treatment, may cause a flulike reaction with elevated body temperature. Managing and reducing these side effects with acetaminophen, NSAIDs, or low-dose oral steroids will ameliorate the disabling symptoms associated with this phenomenon. Recent research evidence suggests that pentoxifylline may be effective in reducing this disabling feature of an important MS therapy (5).

Although MS requires specialized and specialty interventions, primary care services are essential for risk identification, case finding, preventative care, and education, with the goal of wellness. The advanced practice nurse (clinical nurse specialist or nurse practitioner) or physician assistant is finding a valuable niche in the care of the chronically ill patients, and it is anticipated that this role will be strengthened for MS care in during the new millennium.

REFERENCES

1. Paty DW, Ebers GC. Clinical Features in Multiple Sclerosis. In: Paty DW, Ebers GC, eds. *Multiple Sclerosis*. Philadelphia: FA Davis; 1998:135–191.

2. Hoole A, Pickard CG, Ouimette R, et al. *Patient Care Guidelines for Nurse Practitioners*. Philadelphia: JB Lippincott; 1999:45–50.

3. Coyle PK. Multiple sclerosis. In: Kaplan PK, ed. *Neurologic Disease in Women*. New York: Demos Medical Publishing; 1998:251–264.

4. Paty DW, Ebers GC. Clinical features in multiple sclerosis. In: Paty DW, Ebers GC, eds. *Multiple Sclerosis*. Philadelphia: FA Davis; 1998:145–150.

5. Munschauer FE, Kinkel RP. Managing side effects of interferon-beta in patients with relapsing-remitting multiple sclerosis. *Clin Ther*. 1997;19(5):883–893.

CHAPTER 4

The Evolution of Disease Management

Amy Perrin Ross

In recent years, many advances have been made in the understanding and management of multiple sclerosis (MS). Since 1993, four injectable therapies have been approved in the United States by the Food and Drug Administration (FDA): interferon beta-1a (Avonex), interferon beta-1b (Betaseron), and glatiramer acetate (Copaxone), and interferon beta-1a (Rebif) for the treatment of relapsing-remitting multiple sclerosis (RRMS). Another therapy that reentered the MS care paradigm in 2006 is natalizumab (Tysabri), which is given intravenously (IV) every four weeks. These treatments present MS patients and their families with new challenges, including self-injection keeping infusion appointments, and the management of side effects. The nurse plays a pivotal role in patient and family education to optimize treatment with MS therapies.

Injectable Therapy Development

In the 1980s, researchers began studying interferons as a possible treatment for people with MS. It was thought that, because intercurrent viral infections were thought to trigger new attacks of MS, beta-interferons might have an immuno-modulating effect on this process. Interferons are naturally occurring proteins that help regulate the immune system. Interferon-beta binds to specific surface receptors, and it is believed to have antagonistic effects on interferon-gamma and tumor necrosis factor-alpha (TNF-a). The result of this activity is to inhibit the expression of major histocompatibility complex (MHC) class II molecules, which are necessary for T-cell antigen recognition. In addition, interferon beta downregulates expression of adhesion molecules necessary for T-cell migration into the central nervous system (CNS). Interferons are believed to inhibit matrix metalloproteinase (MMP) production that contributes to the disruption of the cellular matrix of the endothelial layer of the blood–brain barrier. In addition, interferon beta is also thought to increase suppressor T-cell activity and increase the activity of interleukin (IL)-10, a regulatory cytokine that is necessary to reduce inflammation.

Interferon Beta-1b (Betaseron)

In 1988, a multicenter, double-blind, placebo-controlled trial was conducted using interferon beta-1b. The study observed 379 patients with RRMS over a 2-year period. Patients were given placebo, 0.05 mg, or 0.25 mg of interferon beta-1b subcutaneously (SC) every other day. The primary outcome measures in the trial were frequency of exacerbation and percentage who were exacerbation-free. In the 2-year analysis there was a 31% reduction in annual exacerbation rate (1). Twenty-five% of patients in the interferon beta-1b group and 16% in the placebo group were exacerbation-free at the 2-year time point. These differences were statistically significant.

Annual magnetic resonance imaging (MRI) scans were performed in 327 of the 379 patients in the study, and 52 patients underwent MRI scans every 6 weeks to evaluate disease activity. The MRI data indicated a significant reduction in disease activity. Expanded disability status scale (EDSS) scores were also evaluated. In this clinical trial, EDSS scores ranged from 0 to 5.5 at baseline and did not significantly change in either the placebo group or the interferon beta-1b group. As a result, the impact of interferon beta-1b on disability could not be evaluated in this trial. Currently, 16-year follow-up data are available on the original cohort of patients in the pivotal trial.

In 1993, the FDA evaluated the results of this pivotal trial and approved interferon beta-1b (Betaseron) for the treatment of RRMS. Betaseron is available in the United States in single-use vials containing 0.25 mg (8 million international units [IU]) of interferon beta-1b. To administer the drug, the patient or caregiver attaches a vial adapter to vial of Betaseron. The next step is to connect a syringe of sodium chloride diluent. All are supplied in a single unit packet for each injection. The diluent is injected into the vial of interferon beta-1b, and the solution is then gently swirled, not shaken. Once dissolved, 1 mL of reconstituted solution is drawn into the sterile syringe. The solution is injected SC every other day. Many patients are taught to slowly increase the dose of the drug when starting Betaseron. A common titration schedule is to inject one-fourth dose for the first 2 weeks followed by half the dose for the next 2 weeks. At the end of the first month, most patients are able to tolerate the full dose with minimal flu-like side effects. An automatic injector device, called the Betaject 3, is available free of charge from the manufacturer and is often used to assist patients with injection technique. Common injection sites include the abdomen, hips, thighs, and arms.

Side effects seen with Betaseron include injection-site reactions and flu-like symptoms. Reddened, hardened areas in the injection sites may develop, and bruising sometimes occurs. Patients should be encouraged to rotate injection sites to reduce complications in one area. Some patients prefer to warm the injection site before injection to relax and increase blood flow to the area. Application of ice to the injection site may also be done but can lead to an increase in injection site reactions due to vasoconstriction in the area. In severe cases, patients may develop skin breakdown and necrosis at the injection sites. A wound management consultation may be necessary to address these more extreme complications.

Some patients also experience flu-like side effects, including fever, chills, fatigue, myalgia, and malaise particularly when starting therapy. These symptoms commonly occur within 24 hours after injection and tend to lessen over time when remaining on treatment. Headache, dizziness, and pain have also been reported side effects. Depression, which is common in people with MS, can be significant at the time patients are starting disease-modifying therapy. Patients with evidence of depression should be appropriately managed before the initiation of therapy.

Interferon Beta-1a (Avonex)

The results of a clinical trial of interferon beta-1a were published by Jacobs and coworkers (2). This pivotal trial was conducted at four MS research centers in the United States. The purpose of the study was to determine whether interferon beta-1a could slow neurologic disability in relapsing MS. A cohort of 301 people with RRMS were randomized in the double-blind, placebo-controlled study. They were given interferon beta-1a (0.25 μg) or placebo by intramuscular (IM) injection once weekly. The primary outcome variable was time to onset of sustained disability, defined as a worsening from baseline by at least one point on the EDSS that persisted at least 6 months. Baseline EDSS scores for inclusion in the trial were between 1.0 and 3.5.

The study showed a significant delay in the time to sustained EDSS progression. The patients treated with interferon beta-1a also had significantly fewer exacerbations and significantly fewer numbers and volume of brain lesions on MRI. In May 1996, the FDA evaluated the results of this trial and approved interferon beta-1a (Avonex) for treatment of relapsing forms of MS. Avonex is available in the United States in single-use vials containing 6.6 million IU (33 µg) of interferon beta-1a or a single prefilled syringe.

To use the powder form of the drug, the patient or care partner first attaches a micropin (vial access pin) to the syringe supplied in the Avonex injection kit. This is then inserted into a vial of diluent (sterile water), which is also supplied; 1.1 mL of diluent is withdrawn and then injected into the vial of lyophilized powder. This vial is then gently swirled until dissolved. Once dissolved, 1 mL of the reconstituted solution is drawn into the syringe. The micropin is removed, and the needle is placed on the syringe for injection. When using the prefilled syringe, the patient is instructed to check the contents of the syringe to see if it is clear. If it is cloudy, it is suggested that the syringe be discarded and another used in its place. There should be 0.5 mL of fluid and an air bubble in the syringe. The patient is instructed to remove the cap and place the 1¼- inch 23-gauge needle on the end of the syringe. The solution is injected IM once per week.

Side effects include headache and flu-like symptoms. Acetaminophen or another nonsteroidal anti-inflammatory (NSAID) is usually recommended before the injection and every 4 hours after for the first 24 hours to reduce side effects. Some patients prefer to ice the injection site briefly before injection to numb the area. Because Avonex is administered as an IM injection, injection site skin reactions are less common than those using SC techniques.

Interferon Beta 1-a (Rebif)

Goodkin (3) published the results of a study of a multicenter clinical trial of interferon beta-1a (Rebif). Rebif was injected in doses of 22 mL or 44 µg SC three times a week. People with a broad range of disability were studied. There were significant reductions in relapse rate, and a significant number of patients had no relapses during the study.

Two pivotal trials evaluating Rebif in RRMS were conducted. The first trial, PRISMS, compared Rebif 22 µg three times weekly, Rebif 44 µg three times weekly, and placebo injections. This trial was conducted in 22 centers in nine countries over 2 years. The results of the trial showed that Rebif significantly reduced MS exacerbations, reduced T2 active lesions, and resulted in more patients being relapse free at the end of 2 years. At the end of the 2-year double-blind placebo-controlled study, patients who were receiving placebo were re-randomized to Rebif 22 µg or 44 µg. The blinding process remained intact. Patients in the trial were then evaluated over the next 2 years. The results of that analysis showed that there was a significantly lower relapse rate over 4 years in those originally randomized to Rebif, particularly Rebif 44 µg. In patients who were on placebo for the first 2 years and then re-randomized to Rebif 44 µg, a significantly lower relapse rate also was noted. Rebif 44 µg given over 4 years also significantly delayed the confirmed progression of disability.

The patients were also evaluated in long-term follow-up at 6 and 8 years. The 6-year follow-up evaluated long-term safety and the 8 year follow-up provided a retrospective and prospective observation of relapses, disability, and MRI endpoints. Relapse rates were lowest in those treated with Rebif from the start. Those on Rebif 44 µg from the beginning of the trial also had the most favorable disability outcomes.

The second pivotal trial evaluating Rebif was the EVIDENCE trial. This was a head-to-head, randomized, open-label, evaluator-blinded comparison of Rebif 44 µg with Avonex 30 µg in patients with RRMS. This trial was required by the U.S. FDA in order for Rebif to enter the U.S. market before the Orphan Drug legislation protection expired for Avonex. The primary end-point of this trial was the proportion of relapse-free patients at 24 weeks. Additional end-point measurements were obtained at 48 weeks. At 72 weeks, those patients initially on Avonex were allowed to cross over to Rebif 44 µg. Results showed that Rebif reduced the risk of relapse by 30% over Avonex at 24 weeks. The number of T2 active lesions was also lower in the Rebif treated group over the length of the trial. Those patients who were originally randomized to Avonex and later crossed over to Rebif saw a 50% decrease in their annualized relapse rates.

Rebif was approved for use in the United States in relapsing forms of MS in 2001. Rebif comes in a prefilled syringe containing 22 µg or 44 µg. A titration pack also is available that contains six syringes of 8.8 µg of Rebif and six syringes of 22 µg. Rebif is injected SC three times a week. The patient typically begins with the 8.8-µg dose three times weekly for the first 2 weeks, and then increases the dose to the 22 µg of Rebif for the next 2 weeks. At the end of the first month most patients are typically ready to increase to the 44 µg dose of Rebif. The Rebiject 2 device, an automatic injector, is also provided to the patient by the manufacturer.

As with Betaseron, side effects seen with Rebif include injection site reactions and flu-like symptoms. Discomfort, as well as reddened, hardened areas in the injection sites may develop, and bruising sometimes occurs. Patients should be encouraged to rotate injection sites to reduce complications in one area. Some patients prefer to warm the injection site before injection to relax and increase blood flow to the area. Many patients find it helpful to take their injection after a warm shower. They are usually more relaxed, and the skin is clean. Application of ice to the injection site may also be done, but can lead to an increase in injection site reactions due to vasoconstriction in the area. Rarely, severe reactions may include development of skin breakdown with necrosis at the injection sites. A wound management consultation may be necessary to address these more extreme complications.

Some patients also experience flu-like side effects, including fever, chills, fatigue, myalgia, and malaise. Titration of the dose of Rebif has significantly reduced the frequency and severity of the flu-like symptoms in many patients. Nonsteroidal anti-inflammatory medications such as acetaminophen or ibuprofen are also helpful in minimizing these side effects. These symptoms commonly occur within 24 hours after injection and tend to lessen over time. Headache, dizziness, and pain have also been reported side effects. As stated earlier, depression, which is common in people with MS, can be significant at the time when patients are starting disease-modifying therapy. Patients with evidence of depression should be appropriately managed before the initiation of therapy.

Glatiramer Acetate

Glatiramer acetate (Copaxone) is a synthetic polypeptide that is similar in structure to normal myelin. It's original development was an effort to provide a synthetic antigen that would induce the animal model of MS, experimental allergic encephalomyelitis (EAE). However, during the early development, it was found to reduce the occurrence and severity of EAE. Although its exact mechanism of action is unclear, it is thought to interfere with antigen presentation by MHC class II molecules. Glatiramer acetate is also thought to induce myelin-specific suppressor T cells and cytokines that regulate immune responses to myelin antigens. These mechanisms of action are thought to be different from those of either interferon beta-1a or interferon beta-1b.

Johnson and coworkers (4) published the result of a pivotal trial of Copaxone in 11 U.S. medical centers. This study evaluated 251 MS patients with EDSS scores of 0 to 5. The primary end-point of the trial was to measure the effect of the drug on the reduction of exacerbation rate. Secondary end-points included evaluating whether the drug slowed progression and documenting any MRI changes. A 29% reduction of exacerbations occurred in the Copaxone group compared with placebo. Those patients with lower EDSS scores showed greater reductions in exacerbations. The clinical trial results also showed a trend toward slowing disability, but the results were not statistically significant. This trial did not have an MRI component. In April 1997, the FDA evaluated the results of the glatiramer acetate trials and approved Copaxone for the treatment of ambulatory patients with mild to moderate relapsing MS. A later, additional trial was done in European and Canadian sites to evaluate the effect on MRI. This was an 18-month trial; 9 months blinded and 9 months open-label. Copaxone was found to reduce new MRI lesions by approximately 30% in this trial.

Copaxone is available in the United States in single-use prefilled syringes containing 20 mg of glatiramer acetate. To administer, the patient or care partner uses the sterile syringe to inject or may insert the syringe into the automatic injector device that is supplied. The solution is injected SC every day. Patients are encouraged to rotate injection sites daily to avoid overuse of one area.

Flu-like side effects are uncommon because Copaxone, unlike interferons, does not induce a rise in body temperature. Some patients experience injection site reactions, including discomfort; hardened, reddened areas; and occasional bruising. Lipoatrophy, a significant dimpling of the skin, is seen in some of the more severe cases, supporting the need for vigilant injection site rotation. Injection site pain was reported in 73% of patients in the clinical trial, and 66% reported injection site erythema. Approximately 10% of MS patients in the Copaxone clinical trial experienced an immediate postinjection reaction. Such reactions could include flushing, anxiety, palpitations, shortness of breath, dyspnea, and chest pain. The symptoms were transient and resolved without treatment. These reactions occurred after several months on therapy and have no known lasting effects. Patients should be educated about the possibility of such reactions to avoid unnecessary anxiety.

Natalizumab (Tysabri)

Natalizumab is a monoclonal antibody that binds to alpha-4-integrin on the surface of all leukocytes except neutrophils, and inhibits the alpha-4–mediated adhesion of leukocytes to their counter-receptors. The receptors for the alpha-4 family of integrins include vascular cell adhesion molecule (VCAM)-1 which is expressed on activated vascular cell endothelium. Disruption of these molecular interactions prevents transmigration of leukocytes across the endothelium into inflamed parenchymal tissue. Tysabri may further act to inhibit the interaction of alpha-4–expressing leukocytes with their ligands in the extracellular matrix and on parenchymal cells, thereby inhibiting the further recruitment and inflammatory activity of activated immune cells.

Natalizumab was evaluated in two randomized, double-blind, placebo-controlled trials in patients with MS. The first trial was the AFFIRM study, which evaluated 300 mg natalizumab IV every 28 days versus placebo in patient who had not received any interferon beta or glatiramer acetate for at least 6 months. 94% of the subjects had never received either of those treatments. The median age was 37, with a median disease duration of 5 years. Patients were randomized in a 2:1 ratio, with more patients receiving natalizumab than placebo. The second trial was the SENTINAL trial. In this trial, patients who had one or more relapses while on treatment with Avonex during the year prior to study entry were enrolled. The medial age was 39, with a median disease duration of 7 years. Patients were evenly randomized to receive 300 mg of natalizumab or placebo IV every 28 days for up to 28 months, in addition to their weekly Avonex injections.

The primary end-point at 2 years was time to onset of sustained increase in disability, defined as an increase of at least 1-point on the EDSS from baseline $\geq .0\ 1$ that was sustained for 12 weeks, or at least a 1.5-point increase on the EDSS from a baseline of 0.

In the AFFIRM trial, the annualized relapse rate reduction was 67%. Significant reductions also occurred in T2 hyperintense lesions and gadolinium (Gd)-enhancing lesions on MRI. In the SENTINAL trial, the relative risk reduction of the annualized relapse rate was 56%, with significant effects on MRI parameters as well.

In November 2004, the FDA approved Tysabri for use in the treatment of relapsing forms of MS. In February 2005, however, the drug was voluntarily recalled from the market due to three cases of progressive multifocal leukoencephalopathy (PML) in patients. PML is an opportunistic infection caused by the JC virus that typically occurs in immunocompromised patients. Two cases occurred in the 1,869 patients treated for MS. The third case of PML occurred in a patient being treated for Crohn'sdisease. An extensive safety evaluation followed the withdrawal of natalizumab. In July 2006, Tysabri was reintroduced to the open market under a restricted access program called TOUCH. Patients, prescribers, pharmacists, and infusion centers, as well as nurses infusing Tysabri must be registered in this program. To enroll in the TOUCH program, both the prescribers and the patients are required to understand the risks of treatment with Tysabri, including PML and other opportunistic infections. Because of the associated risks, Tysabri is generally recommended for patients who have had an inadequate response to, or are unable to tolerate currently available MS therapies. As in the clinical trials, 300 mg of Tysabri is administered IV every 28 days.

Therapies in Clinical Trials

Currently, numerous therapies are in various stages of research clinical trials. *Rituximab* is a monoclonal antibody that depletes B cells by binding to CD20 on the cell surface and initiating cytolytic and cytotoxic pathways. Rituximab is given as an IV infusion at various intervals, depending on the trial. Currently, two trials are ongoing: one evaluating the use of rituximab in RRMS patients, the other evaluating the use of rituximab in primary progressive patients. In a small trial of patients with neuromyelitis optica or progressive relapsing myelitis, all patients remained relapse-free for an average of 6 months.

Cladribine is a purine analog that acts by disrupting the proliferation of monocytes and lymphocytes involved in the pathologic process of MS. A 12-month randomized placebo-controlled study was conducted to evaluate the safety and efficacy of cladribine in 159 patients with progressive MS. No delay in disease progression was observed; however, cladribine produced and sustained significant reductions in the number and volume of Gd-enhanced T1 brain lesions. The T2 lesion load was also reduced. A Phase III trial with 1,200 patients is currently in the final planning stages to evaluate the use of oral cladribine in RRMS patients.

Laquinimod is an orally active immunoregulatory drug that does not have immunosuppressive properties. In a Phase II trial, patients treated with oral laquinimod 0.3 mg three times daily for up to 6 months experienced a significant reduction of 44% in active lesions on MRI compared with placebo. A Phase IIb trial is currently aimed at evaluating the benefit of daily doses of oral laquinimod at 0.3 mg and 0.6 mg versus placebo.

Teriflunomide is an oral dihydro-orotate dehydrogenase inhibitor that has been tested in a 36-week Phase II trial in 179 patients with clinically definite MS. Patients treated with teriflunomide had significantly fewer T1 Gd-enhancing lesions and new T2 lesions compared with the placebo group. In addition, significantly fewer patients treated with teriflunomide 14 mg experienced disease progression, compared to patients with placebo. Currently 870 RRMS patients are being recruited for a Phase III trial.

Another oral immunomodulator, *FTY720*, binds to the sphingosine-1-phosphate receptor on T and B cells and inhibits their release from the lymph nodes. FTY720 is currently in Phase III trials following a 6-month Phase II study involving 281 patients with relapsing MS in which patients treated with FTY720 experienced a reduction in relapse rate of approximately 55% compared with placebo.

Daclizumab is humanized monoclonal antibody against CD25, which is expressed on activated T cells. It is currently approved for the prevention of renal transplant rejection. The use of daclizumab as add-on therapy with interferon beta was investigated in patients with RRMS or secondary-progressive MS (SPMS) who did not respond to interferon beta alone. Daclizumab was administered IV at a dose of 1 mg/kg. The second dose was given 2 weeks after the first, with each succeeding dose administered at 4-week intervals. A total of seven infusions was administered. The number of new contrast-enhancing lesions and total contrast-enhancing lesions was reduced 78% and 70%, respectively, compared to baseline. Patients with RRMS who have failed interferon-beta therapy are currently being recruited into a Phase II open-label trial to assess the use of daclizumab in the treatment of MS.

Alemtuzumab (Campath) is a humanized monoclonal antibody that binds to CD52, which is present on all B and T lymphocytes, and the majority of monocytes, macrophages, and natural killer cells. During an 18-month trial involving 25 patients with SPMS, patients with Gd-enhancing lesions during a 3-month prestudy period were treated with a single-pulse course (20 mg IV daily infusion over 3–4 hours for five consecutive days) of alemtuzumab. They were followed with MRI monthly until 6 months post-treatment, then monthly from 12 to 18 months. The mean number and volume of Gd-enhancing lesions were markedly reduced following treatment with alemtuzumab, compared with pretreatment values. Discussion regarding further trials of alemtuzumab are ongoing.

Patient Education and the Role of the Nurse

Nursing scholar Virginia Henderson (5) said, "Nursing is primarily assisting individuals with those activities contributing to health or its recovery that they perform unaided when they have the necessary strength, will or knowledge; nursing also helps individuals carry out prescribed therapy." These statements clearly identify the role of the nurse in assisting MS patients with injectable therapies. Patient education has been described as recognizing the patient's right to choose her future and willingly sharing knowledge with her (6). In the role of educator, the nurse contributes to the process of influencing behavior and producing the knowledge and skills to maintain and improve health.

The process of patient education begins with assessment. A comprehensive assessment can provide the groundwork for a teaching plan. The assessment of a patient and family living with MS begins with evaluation of their knowledge about the disease and its treatment. The patient may have encountered many sources of information about the disease, including healthcare professionals, the National Multiple Sclerosis Society (NMSS), the Multiple Sclerosis Society of America (MSAA), other people with MS, printed material from sources such as the public library or pharmaceutical companies, and the Internet. The nurse must assess the patient's sources of knowledge and update that knowledge as necessary. Patients often have misconceptions about the disease and treatment options that must be corrected before an effective teaching plan can begin. Another key aspect of assessment is that of the patient's beliefs and values about healthcare and life in general. In our culturally diverse society, the nurse must be increasingly aware of the role these beliefs and values play in the patient's life.

The role of the nurse in patient and family education about injectable therapies often also involves the choice of an injectable therapy. Several key issues to be addressed when making a choice include physical limitations, lifestyle issues, and social support. Physical limitations that must be considered include vision changes, weakness, cognitive changes, numbness, and tremor in the upper extremities. Patients with these limitations often must rely solely on a care partner for assistance. The schedule and availability of a care partner should be evaluated. In some cases, multiple care partners such as family members, neighbors, and friends can be involved. It is important for the patient to realistically evaluate available options before choosing a type of injectable therapy.

Once an injectable therapy has been chosen, the nurse should assess the patient's and family's readiness to learn the self-injection process. Key issues to evaluate include any previous experiences with injections; understanding of how the medication is prepared; and fears such as pain, injection in the wrong area, and needle phobia. These issues may require additional time and discussion before self-injection teaching can begin. Each of the currently available injectable therapies for MS comes with injection teaching booklets and videos to help address some of these issues. Patients are encouraged to review the written materials and videos at home before the teaching session. They should be instructed to take notes and write down their questions before teaching to make the process as smooth as possible. Care partners are also often fearful of making mistakes with the injection and causing pain or inflicting harm. Discussing these issues before injection training will also help to ensure a successful training session. Adult education includes and builds on the experiences of the learner. If the patient or care partner has had negative experiences with injections in the past, these experiences should be openly discussed to avoid problems with future injections.

Lawler (7) noted that adult education is designed to empower the participant. People with MS may feel a sense of empowerment over the disease by taking control of their lives with injectable therapies. Rather than viewing injectable therapy as one more thing that MS has forced them to do, they can be encouraged to look at self-injection as a way of taking control of their daily lives.

Another key element in the self-injection teaching process is the assessment of the best way to conduct the teaching. Some patients and care partners will need intensive one-on-one sessions to accomplish the goal, whereas others will benefit from a group teaching session. Some patients and care partners find support in other members of the group who are experiencing the same thoughts and fears. Teaching sessions may be held in the office or home. Regardless of the type of initial teaching session, follow-up is also important for successful teaching. Nurses may elect to call the patient before or after the next injection to evaluate her understanding of self-injection. Some patients may need to be "walked through" the process again on the phone before the subsequent injection. Even if the patient does well with the initial teaching session, a follow-up phone call in the weeks after the teaching session can reassure the patient about self-injection and answer any questions that may have arisen.

Once the patient has begun the process of self-injection, the nurse must assess adherence to therapy. Problems with adherence to therapy are well documented and estimated to be approximately 50%. Because MS is a chronic disease, the issue of adherence with therapy is a major one. Its unpredictable nature may lead to changes in physical ability, cognitive impairment, or depression, all of which can impact adherence. Adherence can be defined as the active, voluntary, and collaborative involvement of the patient in an acceptable course of behavior that results in a desired outcome (8). Nurses must assess potential barriers that contribute to nonadherence. These include physical ability, knowledge deficits, and cognitive and psychological changes. Care partners can support the patient and reinforce learning on an ongoing basis. Establishing a good nurse–patient relationship can also provide support for the patient. Home care nurses, social workers, physical therapists, occupational therapists, and family and friends can provide additional support that can promote adherence. Pharmaceutical company–funded patient support programs may also help address financial concerns that affect adherence. Patient expectations are well known to affect adherence with injectable therapies. Patients often report that they discontinued an injectable therapy several months after initiation because "I wasn't getting any better." Setting realistic expectations from the start is vital to avoid these pitfalls. Patients should be taught that these therapies are not a cure and are not intended to "make them feel better." Often they initially will feel worse because of side effects. They are far more likely to remain adherent to prescribed regimens if they begin therapy with clear, realistic expectations.

Management of Side Effects

As with most pharmaceutical treatments, the injectable therapies available in the United States and elsewhere for the treatment of MS are associated with side effects (Table 4-1). Munschauer and Kinkel (9) note that there are both class-specific and agent-specific side effects with interferon beta. The most common class-specific side effects are flu-like symptoms, including fever, fatigue, malaise, myalgia, and headaches. These typically begin several hours after injection and usually resolve within 24 hours. These side effects tend to lessen with time and frequently resolve over the first several months on therapy. Subcutaneous injectable therapies also associated with side effects such as injection site reactions. In some cases, there may also be a transient worsening of MS symptoms upon initiation of therapy. Education of the patient about the possibility of side effects before initiation of therapy is essential to ensure adherence. The nurse may also refer the patient to the support programs offered by the manufacturers to assist with the management of side effects.

Flu-like symptoms are most common with interferon beta treatments, and may be seen in more than 50% of patients. Nurses can help patients manage these side effects in a variety of ways. Patients may be encouraged to administer the injection in the evening to reduce the impact on daily activities. Many patients get relief from acetaminophen, 650 mg taken before injection and every 4 hours thereafter for 24 hours. Patients who also experience headache often benefit from NSAIDs such as ibuprofen, aspirin, or naproxen.

Despite these treatments, some patients still experience disabling flu-like side effects. These patients initially may benefit from smaller doses of interferon beta. Patients often begin with 25% to 50% of the full dose, gradually increasing to a full dose as tolerated over several weeks. Oral prednisone, in doses of 10 mg before injection and then every 4 to 6 hours for several more doses, also has proven to be beneficial in reducing side effects. Because most flu-like side effects abate after several months, oral prednisone is usually used only for a short period following therapy initiation. Pentoxifylline, given in 800 mg doses twice a day, has been useful in reducing side effects in patients receiving interferon beta-1b for the first 6 months of therapy. Some patients who also experience disabling fatigue have responded to 100 mg of amantadine twice daily or 200 mg of daily modafinil.

Injection site complications are another type of side effect seen with injectable therapies. Injection site pain may be reduced by applying warm compresses to the area before injection. Some patients also report success with a topical anesthetic. Injection site reactions, including reddened, hardened areas, local

TABLE 4-1
Common Side Effects of *Injectable* Medications

Betaseron and Rebif	Flu-like symptoms, including fever, fatigue, weakness, and myalgias Headache Injection site reactions, including erythema, hard areas, bruising, skin lesions White blood cell abnormalities
Avonex	Flu-like symptoms, including fever, fatigue, weakness, and myalgias Headache Anemia (rare)
Copaxone	Injection site reactions, including erythema, hard areas, bruising Immediate postinjection reaction: chest tightness, anxiety, shortness of breath (rare)

skin lesions, and rare cases of necrotizing skin lesions, can be seen with SC injectables. A constant rotation of injection sites can help keep these reactions to a minimum. The nurse should review injection technique with the patient and care partner to ensure appropriate administration of the medication. Failure to completely dissolve the medication, and injecting a cold solution can also lead to injection site pain and reactions. Patients should be advised to warm the dissolved solution to room temperature to reduce the risk of side effects. Although patients are frequently concerned about bleeding at the injection site, this complication is rare. If the patient aspirates blood before injection, the preparation should be discarded and the patient should be instructed to start the process over with a new mixture. Any discarded drug will be replaced by the manufacturer, so patients should not be concerned about the cost of replacing the dose.

Depression is a common symptom of MS and may be exacerbated at the time patients are deciding to start therapy. Patients should be evaluated and monitored for depression. They should be told about the possibility of worsening existing depression and encouraged to report any symptoms. Depression can be treated with many commonly available antidepressant medications.

Some patients receiving injectable therapies experience insomnia. Changing the timing of injections to earlier in the day is helpful in most cases. Medications such as acetaminophen PM and mild hypnotics are also useful in treating insomnia.

No clinically significant renal, hepatic, or bone marrow abnormalities have been associated with injectable therapies. However, there have been reports of mild leukocyte depression and transaminase elevations in some patients. Complete blood counts and serum chemistries frequently are drawn before therapy initiation. Patients are then monitored while on therapy to identify and correct potential problems early.

In addition to possible injection site reactions, some patients receiving glatiramer acetate experience an immediate postinjection reaction. They report chest tightness, flushing, shortness of breath, and anxiety. These reactions usually last only 10 to 30 minutes and subside without treatment. There have been no known electrocardiographic changes or cardiac sequelae from these reactions. Although such reactions may be frightening, patients should be informed that the reactions are rare. They begin immediately after the injection and can present any time during the course of therapy. They do not occur with each injection, and most patients who have experienced such a reaction have had only one.

Education of the patient and care partner about the possibility of side effects and their potential management is of vital importance to ensure adherence to therapy. Patients who are well prepared initially often deal with side effects much better and are able to continue on therapy for many years.

Patient and Family Support

Many sources of patient and family education and support are available for the MS patient receiving injectable therapies. The nurse who establishes a good nurse–patient relationship is one of the best sources of direct education and support. Each of the pharmaceutical companies also provides company-sponsored support.

- Berlex's Pathways program provides educational materials, training kits for those receiving interferon beta-1b, and a 24-hour hotline staffed by nurses. It also offers injection training from specially trained nurses , a reimbursement hotline, and multiple payment options.
- Serono's MS Lifelines program provides education materials, training kits on Rebif, telephone access to nurses, reimbursement counselors and, in many area of the country, training by nurses who work only with Rebif. In areas where these nurses are not available, nurses can be contracted from national companies to provide injection training.
- Biogen's Avonex Assistance program offers educational materials, a personal journal, an information and reimbursement hotline, a patient starter kit for those receiving Avonex, self-injection training from a national healthcare company, and vouchers for free injection supplies for Avonex patients.
- Teva Neuroscience's Shared Solutions program offers educational materials, an RN counselor (Mon–Fri, 8:00 A.M.–8:00 P.M. EST), insurance department counselors, and self-injection teaching options.

These programs are provided at no cost to the patient, and provide information to any client with MS, whether they are receiving therapy or not. Nurses also often find the hotline numbers very helpful for answering their questions and solving problems. The NMSS has chapters throughout the United States that provide client education, advocacy, and support groups for people with MS and their families. They sponsor educational sessions, provide literature, and in some

TABLE 4-2

Patient Support Programs

Berlex (Betaseron)	"Pathways" 1-800-788-1467 www.betaseron.com
Biogen (Avonex)	"Avonex Alliance" 1-800-456-2255 www.biogen.com
Teva Neuroscience (Copaxone)	"Shared Solutions" 1-800-877-8100 www.tevaneuroscience.com
EMD Serono (Rebif)	MS Lifelines 1-877-447-3243

cases offer peer counseling. Table 4-2 lists the phone numbers of each of the support programs for MS patients.

The Disease Management Advisory Task Force of the NMSS (10) issued a Disease Management Consensus statement about the use of disease-modifying agents. This statement recommends that therapy should be initiated as soon as possible following a definite diagnosis. It is clear from these recommendations that the importance of injectable therapies for MS cannot be underestimated. Multiple sclerosis presents many challenges to the patient, family, care partner, and healthcare professional. Patient education is vital to optimize the treatment of patients with injectable therapies. The nurse is in a unique position to assess patient education needs and design an ongoing teaching plan to support the patient and care partner with MS.

REFERENCES

1. IFNB Multiple Sclerosis Study Group and the University of British Columbia MS/MRI Analysis Group. Interferon beta-1b in the treatment of multiple sclerosis: Final outcome of the randomized controlled trial. *Neurology*. 1995;45:1277–1285.

2. Jacobs LD, Cookfair DL, Rudick RA, et al. Intramuscular interferon beta-1a for disease progression in relapsing multiple sclerosis. The Multiple Sclerosis Collaborative Research Group. *Ann Neurol*. 1996;39:285–294.

3. Goodkin D. Interferon b therapy for multiple sclerosis. *Lancet*. 1998;352(9139):1486–1487.

4. Johnson KP, Brooks BR, Cohen JA, et al. Copolymer 1 reduces relapse rate and improves disability in relapsing-remitting multiple sclerosis: Results of a phase III multicenter, double-blind, placebo-controlled trial. *Neurology*. 1995;45:1268–1276.

5. Henderson V, Nite G. *Principles and Practice of Nursing*, 5th ed. New York: Macmillan; 1960:14.

6. Rankin SH, Stallings KD. *Patient Education: Issues, Principles, Practice*, 2nd ed. Philadelphia: JB Lippincott; 1990:4.

7. Lawler P. Workplace education and the principles and practices of adult education. Unpublished doctoral dissertation, Columbia University, Teachers College, New York, 1988.

8. Multiple Sclerosis Nurse Specialist Consensus Committee. *Multiple Sclerosis: Key Issues in Nursing Management Adherence, Cognitive Function, Quality of Life.* New York: Bioscience. 2004.

9. Munschauer FE, Kinkel RP. Managing side effects of interferon-beta in patients with relapsing-remitting multiple sclerosis. *Intl J Drug Ther.* 1997;19:883–893.

10. MS Disease Management Advisory Task Force. Disease Management Consensus Statement. New York: National Multiple Sclerosis Society, 1998.

CHAPTER 5

Defining and Treating Acute Exacerbations in Multiple Sclerosis

Colleen Harris

Even with advances in disease-modifying therapies, still no treatments are available to eliminate relapses completely, and relapse management remains a significant area in multiple sclerosis (MS) care.

The MS nurse often finds herself at the entry point at a time when a patient seeks help with new symptoms that are interfering with activities of daily living. It is important to understand the appropriate assessment techniques to differentiate between relapses and pseudo-relapses, and to develop management strategies.

What Is a Relapse?

A relapse is defined as the appearance of new neurologic symptoms or worsening of old symptoms of greater than 24 hours' duration and in the absence of fever (1) or other potentially precipitating factors. The individual experiencing the relapse symptoms should not be withdrawing from a previous course of steroids, and there must be a separation of at least 30 days between the resolution of a previous relapse. Usually, relapses evolve over 1 to 7 days, plateau for several weeks, and resolve to some degree over weeks to several months (2).

A clinician diagnosing a true relapse must take a detailed history of relapse symptoms, including the onset, severity, impact on functional abilities, the effect of increased activity, and time of day of symptom occurrence. The anxiety that a disease such as MS provokes often confuses day-to-day symptom fluctuation and overall health changes with symptoms of a relapse. Taking the time to make an accurate diagnosis will limit the long-term consequences of the medications used to manage relapses.

What Is a Psuedorelapse?

A true, acute relapse should not be confused with a pseudorelapse, which is a temporary worsening of symptoms due to a concurrent illness, fever, or infection. General symptoms of infection should be assessed, including fever, chills, muscle and joint aches, and increased fatigue level. A urine culture sho uld be obtained, because urinary tract infections (UTIs) often go undetected in MS and will affect symptoms significantly. In addition, a recent exposure to excessive heat or increased aerobic activity will cause a temporary worsening of symptoms. Waxman determined that the demyelinated nerve is sensitive to heat and will conduct messages with less efficiency with heat exposure (3). During the summer months or in a warm climate, continual heat exposure could lead to long periods of symptom change, and it is very important to rule this out when determining relapse onset.

Relapse Triggers

Infection

Studies have suggested that infections are significant precipitating events for MS relapses. A prospective study by Sibly and colleagues showed that 27% of relapses were preceded by upper respiratory infections (4). This led to the recognized practice of encouraging influenza and pneumonia vaccines in individuals with MS, to avoid immune stimulation and the potential respiratory complication of influenza. Although it has been thought that immunizations could potentially stimulate the immune system and lead to a relapse, studies on the influenza vaccination have failed to show a relation to increased disease activity (5).

In addition there is growing evidence to suggest that UTIs can also precipitate a relapse, and careful attention to good bladder management should be maintained at all times (6). Incomplete bladder emptying occurs in a significant number of individuals with MS and can contribute significantly to kidney and bladder infections. Early intervention with appropriate medications, as well as intermittent catheterization, can minimize bladder infections that may lead to symptom worsening in MS or increased disease activity.

Pregnancy and Nursing

At one time, pregnancy was considered to have a negative impact on MS, and women were not encouraged to have families. Studies have shown that pregnancy does not increase the risk of getting MS (7,8). Some significant research on pregnancy and disease activity in MS has been performed. Researchers demonstrated a 70% decline in relapse activity in the third trimester of pregnancy, and a rebound 70% increase in relapses in the first 3 months postpartum before the attack rate returned to prepregnancy base line.

Breast-feeding has not been linked to increased MS activity (9). One study suggests breast-feeding may decrease relapses in the postpartum period, but this has not been conclusively demonstrated (10). Mothers who nurse their babies must be cautioned about the potential of increased relapse frequency in the early postpartum period and the need to resume their disease-modifying therapies as soon as possible after birth. This may influence their decision to breast-feed their infants because, to date, no evidence exists to validate the safety of these therapies in pregnancy or breast-feeding. This data adds to the growing body of research on the potential role of sex hormones on MS and may pave the way to future hormone-based therapies.

Stress, Surgery, and Trauma

The impact o f anesthesia, surgery, and physical and emotional trauma on MS disease activity has long been a controversial area of exploration. Some studies suggest that anesthesia and surgery (11,12) can lead to increased relapse rate, but prospective studies have failed to prove this conclusively (13). An extensive amount of evidence also exists on the link between increased life stressors and increased activity as well, but academics remain skeptical that there is a true correlation. Anecdotally, many of our patients report stressful life events prior to the onset of relapses and certainly the impact of prolonged unmanaged stress has been a known link to adverse overall health, m aking wellness-focused lifestyle strategies and stress management techniques important in the education of patients.

Heat Exposure

Research on increasing neurologic symptoms following exposure to warm water has long been accepted in the MS world (14). Overall neurologic function in individuals with MS may temporarily deteriorate after exercise, with increased body temperature, and with increased ambient temperature as well. Often these changes can be attributed to an MS relapse. Individuals must be educated on the role of heat and on measures to reduce their core body temperatures. Cool drinks and air conditioning in the summer months can alleviate these symptoms fairly quickly. Patients should also be instructed to take frequent rests while exercising and to be prepared for short periods of increased symptoms after an aerobic workout.

Educating the Patient and Family

The importance of recognizing new MS activity is vital in a changing world of MS therapies, where a major goal is to control the rate and severity of relapses. Individuals must be taught to recognize symptom change and discern if symptom change is part of daily fluctuation or the onset of new disease activity. Often keeping a journal on symptoms and noting the onset, location, and duration of changes can be very helpful to the clinicians managing their care. Eliminating other possible causes of pseudorelapses is also important, and patients should be instructed to rule out infections, especially those involving the urinary tract, as well as viral illnesses. It is also important to allow an adequate amount of time between relapses. Many patients who experience a true relapse will have their symptoms worsen before they get better, and this often is mistaken for a new relapse. Relapses must be separated by at least 30 days to be considered distinct relapses.

It is also vital for the patient and family to keep track of relapses. This will assist the care team in determining if disease-modifying therapies are needed or are being effective. Accurate recording is very helpful, and individuals must also understand that not all relapses are treated. If patients are experiencing mild relapses that are not affecting their activities of daily living, they must understand that medication is not always used in treatment. Rest and time will do as much for a relapse, and repeated exposure to the drugs used to treat relapses (such as steroids) is not warranted. Overuse of steroid treatments and abuse of unproven alternative therapies can have serious consequences. Individuals should be counseled to call their MS nurse or physician when a relapse is significantly impacting their lives. Most patients learn when they need treatment, and knowing the correct resources to contact when they are uncertain can ensure the appropriate treatment at the right time.

A wellness-based life style can also help patients steer clear of some of the known triggers for MS relapses. Eating well and getting adequate amounts of rest will help in the overall health of all body functions, including the immune system. Ensuring a yearly flu shot will help to avoid one of the immune triggers thought to contribute to increased disease activity. Good bladder management and avoidance of other secondary infections are also important for preventative treatment. In a disease that robs patients of so much control, it is rewarding to equip them with knowledge to control those factors that are in their power to manage.

Five disease-modifying therapies are approved for use in MS: Betaseron, Avonex, Rebif, and Tysabri. These agents have been demonstrated, in well-designed placebo-controlled Phase III studies, to reduce the frequency of MS relapses and MS-related magnetic resonance imaging (MRI) activity. These therapies have brought great hope to MS management, but have created a new source of uncertainty for patients. These medications are not curative; when patients who are taking them have a relapse, it can be a significant source of anxiety. Patients and families must start therapy with realistic expectations, and these expectations need to be reinforced constantly by the MS care team. Often, the occurrence of a relapse will provoke anxiety in both the patient and family. Having adequate coaching and support will enable patients to work through this situation and know when concern and treatment change is necessary or when worry is unwarranted.

Treatment of Relapses

Glucocorticoids

Once a true relapse is determined, the decision to treat must be made. If a relapse is severe enough to significantly impact an individual's activities of daily living, treatment with high-dose glucocorticoids either by the oral or intravenous (IV) route is indicated. Glucocorticoids have an anti-inflammatory effect on the inflammation in the central nervous system caused by demyelination. Little evidence suggests that high-dose steroids alter the course of the disease, but they are felt to hasten the resolution of acute relapses (15). Researchers involved in the Optic Neuritis Treatment trial suggested that IV steroids were superior to the oral route for acute optic neuritis (16) and, although expensive, this route remains a popular way to treat relapses in North America MS Centers. A common dose schedule for the IV route is methylprednisolone 1 g/day for 3 to 5 days. This is often followed by an oral prednisone taper. However, high oral doses of prednisone (1,250 mg on alternate or daily dose schedules of 3 to 5 days) have also been used and found to be as safe and effective as the IV route (17,18).

The Multiple Sclerosis Council for Clinical Practice Guidelines has stated that, for treatment of acute relapses, no strong evidence suggests that one type of glucocorticoid is more beneficial than another, nor does route of administration affect outcome (19). Patients receiving glucocorticoids must be appraised of the purpose and expectations of treatment, as well as both the short- and long-term side effects. The outcome of shortening the duration and alleviating relapse symptoms should be emphasized. Short-term side effects include metallic taste, facial flushing, altered appetite, weight gain, stomach upset, restlessness, mood swings, insomnia, and fluid retention. A small percentage of patients may experience psychosis secondary to the administration of steroids, and it is advisable that patients have friends or family monitor them at home during the course of their treatment. Long-term side effects can include cataract formation, gastrointestinal bleeding, osteoporosis, osteonecrosis of the hip, and diabetes. The risk of the occurrence of serious side effects can be reduced by only treating more serious relapses and using brief courses of steroids. Those receiving steroids should also be placed on both calcium and vitamin D supplements. All patients who have received steroid treatment for relapses should be followed on an ongoing basis for potential long-term side eff ects.

Adrenocorticotropic Hormone

Adrenocorticotropic hormone (ACTH) by intramuscular (IM) injection has been used in the past to stimulate the patient's own adrenal cortex to produce cortisol, corticosterone, and aldosterone. Patients have demonstrated variable hormonal and clinical responses to this therapy, and its use clearly declined with the acceptance of both IV and orally administered glucocorticoids (20). Recently, this therapy has reemerged because of shortages of IV methylprednisolone. A purified gel preparation designed for extended release when given by IM injection is now being used in a variety of dose regimens for acute relapses. The side-effect profile of ACTH is similar to both IV and oral glucocorticoids, with the added concerns of site reactions and abscess formation from this method of injection.

Intravenous Immunoglobulin

Intravenous immunoglobulin (IVIg) is also a therapy that rises and falls in favor in the treatment of acute relapses. Case study reports and a pilot study have suggested that this therapy has a role in reversing deficits in relapsing-remitting MS (RRMS) (21). There are several negative prospective studies that have failed to demonstrate the benefit of using IVIg in relapse management (22–24). Cost and supply issues have also limited its wide use, along with the fact that it is a human blood derivative and carries the risk of blood-borne diseases such as hepatitis C. Some clinicians may use it as second-line management of persistent disease activity. Common side effects include headache, nausea, and skin rashes.

Plasmapheresis

Plasmapheresis, the process of separating plasma from the blood, mixing it with other fluids, and retransfusing it, has been investigated for its use in acute relapses of MS over the past two decades. A controlled trial failed to show benefit when plasmapheresis was used along with ACTH and cyclophosphamide for acute attacks (25). The patients in this study were of a mixed variety of severity and MS type, and this prompted a closer look at the utility of this procedure in a population with more active inflammatory disease. A double-blind cross-over Phase II study demonstrated that up to 40% of patients with severe inflammatory-demyelinating events who did not respond to IV corticosteroids demonstrated significant improvement on a course of seven alternate-day plasma exchange treatments (24). This procedure is both invasive and expensive, and it is currently reserved for more catastrophic MS attacks or variants of MS such as neuromyelitis optica.

Rehabilitation

The role of rehabilitation cannot be overlooked in the treatment of relapses. Assistive upper limb devices and mobility aids may be required for incomplete recovery and residual deficits. Often a patient must be educated on energy conservation techniques, because fatigue often intensifies during the relapse period. A growing body of evidence suggests that rehabilitation benefits the person with MS in a variety of outcomes. In addition, the role of the multidisciplinary care team—including the rehabilitation specialist — is recognized as the ideal model of service across the spectrum of MS (26). Following a MS relapse, the patient may be faced with limitations that affect mobility and the ability to maintain regular activities of daily living. Some data suggest that gait re-education (27) and muscular endurance training (28) can be effective in MS and may be of value in restoring function following a relapse. Unfortunately, there is a significant lack of coordinated rehabilitation services throughout the world, and reimbursement for this type of care remains a challenge for most healthcare systems. Ongoing research on therapy outcomes, along with reimbursement advocacy, will remain a necessity in the future.

Nursing Considerations in Relapse Management

Relapses signify a very traumatic time for individuals affected by MS. A relapse can be the beginning of a diagnosis, or a signal that the disease is not stable or that therapy is not effective. This period can provoke uncertainty, anxiety, and depression. The role of a nurse as an educator, counselor, and patient and family advocate is vital. The duties of a nurse at this time can range from being a voice at the end of a telephone line offering support and education, to one of front-line assessment, treatment, or even bed-side care. The needs of the patient are enormous, even in the absence of physical limitations. It is imperative that nurses involved in MS care remain updated on current advances in treatment as well as on strategies that will assist their patients in coping, such as rehabilitation and psychosocial counseling. An MS nurse can empower those affected to navigate through this period and make the necessary adjustments that will help them maintain a good quality of life and a sense of hope in the future.

REFERENCES

1. Poser CM, Paty DW, Scheinberg L, et al. New diagnostic criteria for multiple sclerosis: Guidelines for research protocols. *Ann Neurol.* 1983;13:227–231.

2. Coyle P. Diagnosis and Classification of Inflammatory Demyelinating Disorders. In: Burks J, Johnson K, eds. *Multiple Sclerosis Diagnosis, Medical Management, and Rehabilitation.* New York: Demos; 2000:84.

3. Waxman SG. ed. Clinical course and electrophysiology of multiple sclerosis. *Neurology: Functional Recovery in Neurological Disease.* New York: Raven Press; 1988:157–158.

4. Sibley WA, Bamford CR, Clark K. Clinical viral infections and multiple sclerosis. *Lancet.* 1985;4:1313–1315.

5. Myers LW, Ellison GW, Lucia M, et al. Swine influenza virus vaccination in patients with multiple sclerosis. *J Infect Dis.* 1977;136 (Suppl):546–554.

6. Metz lM, McGuinness SD, Harris CJ. Urinary tract infections may trigger relapse in multiple sclerosis. *Axon.* 1998;19:67–70.

7. Abramsky O. Pregnancy in multiple sclerosis. *Ann Neurol.* 1994;36:S38–S41.

8. Leibowitz U, Antonovsky A, Kats R, Alter M. Does pregnancy increase the risk of multiple sclerosis? *J Neurol Neurosurg Psychiatry.* 1967;30:354–357.

9. Confavreux C Hutchinson M, Hours MM, et al. Rate of pregnancy related relapses in multiple sclerosis. *N Engl J Med.* 1998;339:285–291.

10. Confravreux C, Vukusis S, Adeleine P.et al. Pregnancy and multiple sclerosis (the PRIMS study); 2 year results. *Neurology.* 2001;56:A197.

11. McAlpine D, Compston ND. Some aspects of natural history of disseminated sclerosis. *QJM.* 1952;82:135–167.

12. Siemkowicz E. Multiple sclerosis and surgery. *Anaesthesia.* 1976;31:1211–1216.

13. Bamford CR, Sibley WA, Thies C, et al. Trauma as an etiologic and aggravating factor in multiple sclerosis. *Can J Neurol Sci.* 1981;31:1229–1234.

14. Berger JR, Sheremata WA. Persistent neurological deficits precipitated by hot bath test in multiple sclerosis. *JAMA.* 1983;249:1751–1753.

15. Goodkin DE, Kinkel R, Weinstock-Guttman B, et al. A phase II study of IV methylprednisolone in secondary progressive multiple sclerosis. *Neurology.* 1998;51:239–245.

16. Beck RW, Cleary PA, Trobe JD, et al. The effect of corticosteroids for acute optic neuritis on the subsequent development of multiple sclerosis. The Optic Neuritis Study Group. *N Engl J Med.* 1993;329:1764–1769.

17. Metz LM, Sabuda D, Hilsden RJ, et al. Gastric tolerance of high dose pulse oral prednisone in multiple sclerosis. *Neurology.* 1999;53:2093–2096.

18. Morrow SA, Stoian CA, Dmitrovic J, et al. The bioavailability of methylprednisolone and oral prednisone in multiple sclerosis. *Neurology.* 2004;63:1079–1080.

19. Multiple Sclerosis Council for Clinical Practice Guidelines. *Disease Modifying Therapies in Multiple Sclerosis: Evidence Based Management Strategies for Disease Modifying Therapies in Multiple Sclerosis.* Washington, DC: Paralyzed Veterans of America; 2001:12–13.

20. Snyder BD, Lakatua DJ, Doe RP. ACTH-induced cortisol production in multiple sclerosis. *Acta Neurol.* 1981;10:388–389.

21. Van Engelen BG, Hommes OR, Pinckers A, et al. Improved vision after intravenous immunoglobulin in stable demyelinating optic neuritis. *Ann Neurol.* 1992;32:834–835.

22. Stangel M, Boegner F, Klatt CH, et al. Placebo controlled pilot trial to study the remyelinating potential of intravenous immunoglobulins in multiple sclerosis. *J Neurol Neurosurg Psychiatry.* 2000;68:89–92.

23. Noseworthy JH, O'Brien PC, Weinshenker BG, et al. IV immunoglobulin does not reverse established weakness in MS. *Neurology.* 2000;55:1135–1143.

24. Noseworthy JH, O'Brien C, Petterson TM, et al. A randomized trial of intravenous immunoglobulin in inflammatory demyelinating optic neuritis. *Neurology.* 2001;56:1514–1522.

25. Weiner HL, Dau PC, Khatri BO, et al. Double blind study of true vs sham plasma exchange in patients treated with immunosuppression for acute attacks of multiple sclerosis. *Neurology.* 1989;39:1143–1149.

26. Harris C, Costello K, Halper J, et al. Consortium of multiple sclerosis centers recommendations for care of those affected by multiple sclerosis. *Int J MS Care.* 2003;5:67–78.

27. Lord SE, Wade DT, Halligan PW. A comparison of two physiotherapy treatment approaches to improve walking in multiple sclerosis: A pilot randomized controlled study. *Clin Rehabil.* 1998;12:477–486.

28. Gehlsen GM, Grinsby SA, Winant DM. Effects of an aquatic fitness program on muscular strength and endurance of patients with multiple sclerosis. *Phys Ther.* 1984;64:653–657.

CHAPTER 6

Infusion Therapies in Multiple Sclerosis: Nursing Implications

June Halper and Marie A. Namey

O ver the past three decades, multiple sclerosis (MS) therapies have ranged from oral medications, to intramuscular (IM) injections (adrenocorticotropic hormone [ACTH] during the 1980s, Avonex during the 1990s), to infusion therapies for acute relapses during the 1980s, to chemotherapy (cyclophosphamide) for worsening disease. This potpourri of treatments was enhanced by the approval of self-injectable medications during the 1990s. Thus the focus on infusions for MS shifted to a recent re-emphasis of their use in MS care. This may not diminish as new and emerging research demonstrates the benefits of infusible medications.

The use of infusion therapies in MS is associated with numerous challenges, not the least of which are those issues important to infusion nurses. Nurses who specialize in infusions generally are familiar with infectious diseases, various types of cancers, and conditions that result in hematologic disorders. Multiple sclerosis, a neurologic disease with widespread physical, emotional, and psychosocial implications, poses specific challenges to the infusion nurse. These include the physical, learning, and emotional needs related to the dynamic condition that defines as MS. So, in addition to the appropriate evaluation and monitoring of patients with MS, training in administration of MS therapies, managing side effects of these MS treatments, and patient scheduling and office logistics, infusion nurses also require information and support themselves. The MS nurse must be advised of each patient's needs, the type of medication that has been prescribed, its side-effects, and the rationale for therapy.

Multiple Sclerosis Therapies Administered by Infusion

Similar to certain types of cancers, autoimmune deficiencies, and specific infections, many newer MS treatments are administered by infusion. Therapies that have traditionally been given intravenously (IV) include corticosteroids, chemotherapeutic agents such as mitoxantrone and cyclophosphamide, immunoglobulin, and natalizumab.[a] Based on a consensus meeting coordinated by the International Organization of MS Nurses, it was suggested that, before the start of each infusion, a preinfusion checklist should be completed (Table 6-1), with the prescriber notified prior to the start of infusion if any of the characteristics on the checklist are present (1).

Corticosteroids

Corticosteroids are potent anti-inflammatory agents (Table 6-2). Of the two corticosteroids frequently used in MS—methylprednisolone and dexamethasone—only the former is approved by the U.S. Food and Drug Administration

TABLE 6-1
Pre-Infusion Checklist

The infusion nurse should contact the prescriber prior to start of the infusion if any of the following are present:

Characteristic	≥
Pregnancy or breast-feeding	
Elevated body temperature	
Untreated infection (UTI, URI)	
Vaccine within the past 2 weeks	
Abnormal vital signs (low or elevated blood pressure, irregular pulse, tachycardia)	
Skin changes (rash, pressure ulcer)	
Diabetes	
Other medical complaints (chest pain, edema, shortness of breath)	

UTI, urinary tract infection; URI, upper respiratory infection.

---

[a] Although used in MS, cyclophosphamide and immunoglobulin are not considered approved MS therapies.

TABLE 6-2
Corticosteroids

Rationale for use	Potent anti-inflammatory agents that can reduce inflammation in the brain and spinal cord
Dose	Methylprednisolone: 1 g/day IV every day for 3–5 days for relapse
	Dexamethasone: 160–180 mg/day IV every day for 3–5 days for relapse*
	After the 3–5 days, a taper of the oral form of these drugs is common
	Regularly scheduled corticosteroid treatment may be given long term
Benefits	May relieve symptoms and reduce the severity and duration of an MS relapse
	A patient's response to corticosteroids may differ with each attack
Side effects	During infusion: metallic taste in the mouth, flushing, headache, low back pain, and anxiety
	After or between infusions: insomnia, indigestion, heartburn, nausea, fluid retention, mood changes, reduced potassium levels, temporary elevation in blood sugar levels, blood pressure elevation, delayed hives
	Longer-term side effects: osteoporosis, cataracts, irregular menses, decreased resistance to infection, skin changes
Nursing measures to modify side effects	*During infusion:* • Metallic taste: suggest hard candy • Flushing: will dissipate with time (usually a few days after the infusion is complete) • Headache and low back pain: slowing infusion rate and/or an analgesic
	After or between infusions: • Insomnia: over-the-counter (OTC) drugs (Tylenol PM or Benadryl) or a prescription sleep aid • Indigestion/heartburn: OTC gastrointestinal protective agents (Pepcid, Tums) • Fluid retention and swelling: decrease salt intake; drink more fluids • Potassium decrease: eat foods high in potassium (oranges, bananas, potatoes, broccoli) • Mood changes: may require pharmacologic intervention • Temporary elevation in blood sugar levels: a low-sugar diet • Blood pressure elevation: check blood pressure prior to infusion

(Continued)

TABLE 6-2 (Continued)

	• Delayed hives: should be immediately reported to the health care professional
	Longer-term: • Corticosteroid-induced osteoporosis: calcium 1,200–1,500 mg/day with vitamin D
	Administering corticosteroids before noon is recommended to mimic the patient's normal cortisol pattern
Alerts	• Unremitting hypertension • Marked changes in mood (euphoria, irritability, nervousness, restlessness) • Elevated temperature • Abnormally high blood sugar levels

Data used with permission from Decadron phosphate [package insert]. Whithouse Station, NJ: Merck & Co., Inc.; 2001, and methylprednisolone package insert.

*Frequently, oral corticosteroids are used in place of IV administration based on clinician opinion and experience.

(FDA) specifically for use in acute exacerbations of MS (2,3). Corticosteroids may relieve symptoms and reduce the severity and duration of a MS relapse. Although corticosteroids reduce inflammation, recovery from an attack will be determined by the body's ability to heal. A patient's response to corticosteroids may differ with each attack. Sometimes corticosteroids are used on a regularly scheduled basis (pulse therapy) to modify the disease.

Chemotherapeutic Agents

Mitoxantrone (4)

Mitoxantrone is a chemotherapeutic agent FDA-approved for clinically worsening MS (Table 6-3) (3). It is beneficial in MS because it suppresses the number and activity of white blood cells that induce the MS attack in the central nervous system (CNS). Because mitoxantrone can suppress the immune system, those receiving treatment should avoid contact with people who are sick, and should avoid dental procedures for 2 to 3 weeks after each dose. A major limitation of mitoxantrone treatment is that, because of cumulative cardiotoxicity, lifetime use is restricted to 140 mg/m^2. This is most commonly administered in 8 to 12 doses over 2 to 3 years, but may vary.

Cyclophosphamide (6)

Cyclophosphamide is a chemotherapeutic agent that is not FDA-approved for treatment of MS (i.e., it is used *off-label*), although it has been studied since

TABLE 6-3

Mitoxantrone

Rationale for use	Suppression of the activity of white blood cells that induce the MS attack in the CNS
Dose (4)	12 mg/m² IV every 3 months for up to 24 months (with a lifetime maximum allowable dose of 140 mg/m²)
Benefits	May reduce relapse rate and slow progression of disease
Side effects (5)	◆ Blood: decreased resistance to infection, *leukopenia* ◆ Cardiac: cumulative cardiotoxicity, shortness of breath ◆ CNS: increased fatigue ◆ Gastrointestinal: nausea, vomiting, diarrhea ◆ Integumentary: temporary hair thinning, stomatitis, blue-tinted sclera ◆ Endocrine: menstrual irregularities, amenorrhea ◆ Genitourinary: UTI, blue-tinted urine ◆ Senses: blue-tinted tears
Nursing measures	*Prior to each dose:* ◆ Cardiac monitoring (history and physical examination, left ventricular ejection fraction [LVEF], congestive heart failure) ◆ Hematologic monitoring (inform patient of signs of infection, complete blood count and platelets prior to each course and if signs of infection [only infuse if absolute neutrophil count is ≥1,500 cells/mm³]) ◆ Hepatic monitoring (liver function test [do not treat if baseline LVEF <50%]) ◆ Confirm negative pregnancy test/confirm not breast-feeding ◆ Cumulative dose monitoring
	In addition: ◆ Obtain recent height and weight ◆ Instruct patients to eat light meal ◆ Use Angiocath (22-gauge desirable); do not use butterfly needle ◆ Verify blood return before and after infusion ◆ Check frequently for infiltration; if it occurs, no antidote, apply ice, report to health care professional immediately ◆ Inform patients to avoid dental work/surgical procedures for first 2–3 weeks after each treatment ◆ Inform patients to avoid contact with anyone sick for the first 12–14 days after each treatment ◆ Inform patient on importance of postinfusion blood draws and monitoring ◆ Follow standard chemotherapy precautions and personal protective equipment

(Continued)

TABLE 6-3 (Continued)

Alerts (5)	◆ Medication extremely irritating to veins and skin (in the event of contact with skin, rinse with copious amounts of water and observe for irritation) ◆ LVEF <50% or clinically significant reduction ◆ Absolute neutrophil count <1,500 cells/mm³ ◆ Signs/symptoms of infection ◆ Extreme weakness ◆ Infiltration ◆ Receipt of chemotherapy for any other indication

the early 1980s (Table 6-4). Like mitoxantrone, its mechanism of action as a chemotherapeutic agent is suppression of white blood cells.

Immunoglobulins (7)

Immunoglobulins (IVIg or HIGG) are concentrated immune factors that temporarily modify the immune system, although the exact mechanism by which they work in MS is unknown (Table 6-5). Although some patients benefit from immunoglobulin, this medication is not FDA approved for treatment in MS, and it is expensive. Further clinical trials are needed to determine the usefulness of this treatment in MS. Immunoglobulins can be given in a number of different doses and on a number of different schedules. A common dosage is 400 mg/kg once daily for 3 to 5 days. A once-monthly infusion of 0.15 to 0.2 g/kg is also an option. Infusion time can range from 2 to 6 hours or more depending on the patient's dose and overall tolerance.

Natalizumab (8)

Natalizumab was recently FDA approved for the treatment of relapsing forms of MS (Table 6-6). It works differently from any other disease-modifying agent: It is a monoclonal antibody that reduces the movement of active immune cells into the CNS. This reduces inflammation and demyelination in the CNS and slows the worsening of MS. Natalizumab is administered every 4 weeks as a 1-hour infusion.

Three cases of progressive multifocal leukoencephalopathy (PML) have been reported in patients treated with natalizumab for longer than 2 years or who received it intermittently over 18 months (patients were concomitantly exposed to immunomodulators [e.g., interferon beta] or were immunocompromised due to treatment with immunosuppressants [e.g., azathioprine]). It is unclear whether the risk of PML is increased in patients treated with natalizumab in combination with interferon beta compared with natalizumab alone. A comprehensive safety

TABLE 6-4

Cyclophosphamide

Rationale for use	Suppression of the number and activity of white blood cells that induce the MS attack in the CNS
Dose	Varies; adjusted based on number of white blood cells. May be administered by induction (several days in a row) or as pulse therapy (intermittently, usually monthly or every other month)
Benefits	Modest improvement (at best) in patients with progressive MS
Side effects	• Allergy: local histamine reaction (nasal congestion, sneezing, headache) during infusion • Gastrointestinal: nausea and/or vomiting (usually developing after infusion and lasting <24 hours), lack of appetite, mouth sores • Genitourinary: cystitis (including frequent urination), bleeding when voiding, bladder tumors • Endocrine: menstrual irregularities, low sperm count with possible sterility, possible risk to unborn child • Integumentary: hair loss (reversible), skin/nail color changes (reversible) • Blood: decreased resistance to infection, secondary malignancies (in some patients receiving cyclophosphamide for other diseases)
Nursing measures	*Prior to each course:* • Hematologic monitoring (inform patient of signs of infection, complete blood count, and platelets prior to each course and if signs of infection [only infuse if white blood cell count $\geq$1,500 cells/mm^3]) • Pregnancy testing/confirm not breast-feeding • Obtain recent weight
	In addition: • Pre- and postinfusion hydration (postinfusion: 3 L each day for 3 days) • Instruct patients to void after infusion • Instruct patients to eat light meal • Use Angiocath (22-gauge desirable); do not use butterfly needle • Verify blood return before and after infusion • Check frequently for infiltration; if it occurs, no antidote, apply ice, report to health care professional immediately • Urinalysis with cytology yearly; after 3 years, cystoscopy yearly • Inform patients to avoid dental work/surgical procedures for first 2–3 weeks after each treatment • Inform patients to avoid contact with anyone sick for the first 12–14 days after each treatment • Follow standard chemotherapy precautions and personal protective equipment • Advise patients who will be receiving influenza or pneumonia vaccines to do so in the week prior to their infusion (3 weeks after their last infusion)

(Continued)

TABLE 6-4 (Continued)

Alerts	• White blood cell count <1,500 cells/mm³
	• Signs/symptoms of infection
	• Abdominal pain
	• Extreme weakness
	• Receipt of chemotherapy for any other indication

TABLE 6-5
Immunoglobulins

Rationale for use	May temporarily modify the immune system
Dose	Common dosage is 400 mg/kg once daily for 3–5 days for initial course and varies thereafter depending on response
Benefits	May slow the disease process
Side effects	• CNS: anxiety, malaise, fatigue, headache
	• *Musculoskeletal: myalgia, arthralgia, abdominal pain
	• Flu-like: chills*, fever
	• Cardiac: blood pressure changes*
	*Symptoms may be rate related
	• Rare: aseptic meningitis, seizures, acute encephalopathy, hypersensitivity reactions, congestive heart failure, acute renal failure
Nursing measures	*Prior to each course:*
	• Benadryl or Tylenol may be ordered
	• Check vital signs prior to each rate increase, then hourly
	• Monitor closely for signs of hypersensitivity reaction, fluid overload, and congestive heart failure
	In addition:
	• Inform patient that IVIg is a human blood product. Although there is a possibility for infection, the industry screens for viruses and, to date, no known cases of infection from IVIg have been reported in MS patients
	• Assess for history of reaction to blood or blood product
Alerts	• Renal insufficiency
	• History of thrombosis, congestive heart failure, uncontrolled hypertension

TABLE 6-6
Natalizumab

Rationale for use	Reduces the movement of active immune cells into the CNS
Dose	Recommended: 300 mg every 4 weeks administered as a 1-hour infusion
Benefits	Significantly reduces relapses, disability progression, and development of new lesions on MRI

(Continued)

TABLE 6-6 (Continued)

Side effects	*Common:* • General: headache, fatigue, arthralgia, allergic reaction, urinary urgency/frequency, chest discomfort, local bleeding, rigors • Infection: UTI, lower respiratory tract infection, gastroenteritis, vaginitis, tonsillitis • Psychiatric: depression • Gastrointestinal: abdominal discomfort, abnormal liver function test • Skin: rash, dermatitis, pruritus • Menstrual disorders: irregular menstruation/dysmenorrhea, amenorrhea • Neurologic: vertigo
	Serious: • Infections, hypersensitivity reactions (mild, moderate, or severe; anaphylaxis/anaphylactoid), depression, cholelithiasis
Nursing measures	• Prior to starting treatment, the health care professional completes a patient checklist to ensure that the patient meets all requirements for use of natalizumab. • Prior to each infusion, the patient and infusion nurse complete a checklist to screen for symptoms suggestive of PML. • Gently invert the solution to mix completely; do not shake; inspect visually for particulates prior to administration. • Natalizumab is only compatible with normal saline solution and must be used immediately after reconstitution. • Infuse over 1 hour; do not administer as an IV push or bolus injection. • Observe patients during the infusion and for 1 hour after infusion is complete (Angiocath should remain in place in the event rescue medications are needed). • Monitor for signs of hypersensitivity; promptly discontinue the infusion upon first signs/symptoms consistent with a hypersensitivity-type reaction
Alerts	• Hypersensitivity: usually occurs within 2 hours of start of infusion; if hypersensitivity reaction occurs, discontinue administration and consider the possibility of natalizumab antibodies. • PML: obtain MRI scan prior to initiating therapy; prior to each infusion, the patient and infusion nurse complete a checklist to screen for symptoms suggestive of PML; suspend dosing at first signs/symptoms and perform Gd+ brain MRI; cerebrospinal fluid analysis for JC viral DNA may also be useful to confirm a diagnosis of PML. • Immunosuppression: safety and efficacy of natalizumab in combination with antineoplastic or immunosuppressive agents have not been established; concurrent use of these agents with natalizumab may increase the risk of infections, including opportunistic infections (9).

analysis estimated the risk of PML as 1 case per 1,000 patients in 3,116 patients with a mean natalizumab exposure of approximately 18 months (9).

Treatment Challenges Specific to MS

Treatment challenges specific to MS include patient issues (physical, cognitive, and emotional), potential problems with IV access in some patients, and a wide range of psychosocial issues. Mobility problems can prevent a patient from accessing clinical services, including treatment. Other physical symptoms, such as tremor and fatigue, can also impair a patient's ability to adhere to treatment regimens. Bladder dysfunction can be challenging because urinary frequency (a common MS symptom) may interfere with the administration of certain treatments infused over several hours (e.g., immunoglobulins). In addition, bladder dysfun-ction can result in UTIs, with the presence of any type of active infection precluding treatment with corticosteroids, mitoxantrone, or cyclophosphamide. Cognitive problems (including difficulty with learning/remembering new material and sequencing activities) are experienced by approximately half of patients with MS (10,11). Cognitively impaired patients may have difficulty both in remembering to take their medication and in carrying out the multistep procedures of self-injection and self-infusion. Mood changes, including depression, may affect a patient's willingness or ability to adhere to treatment regimens. Because depre ssion is quite common in MS, all patients should routinely be screened, with treatment strategies including psychotherapy and antidepressant medication (12).

Problems with IV access often occur in patients with MS. Poor venous access may be due to poor hydration, scarring of the vein from overuse, decreased neurologic function, and/or decreased muscle tone. Because of IV access issues, it may be recommended that a peripherally inserted central catheter (PICC) line or port be placed prior to exhausting all of a patient's veins.

Due to its wide scope of disease burden, various psychosocial factors are associated with MS, all of which can impede treatment adherence. Social isolation and the stigma associated with MS may have a negative impact on patient adherence. The diagnosis of MS carries with it a life-long emotional impact, and this may impair a patient's motivation or ability to adhere to treatment. A relatively common psychosocial factor in MS is financial in nature. Many patients are expected to take a wide variety of expensive medications and need costly equipment (such as wheelchairs and transfer devices). At the same time, a patient's income may be restricted due to inability to work secondary to physical and/or cognitive deficits. In addition, lack of adequate insurance coverage can interfere with a patient's capacity to adhere to a comprehensive management program (Chapter 7).

Summary

The scope of the MS care team has broadened to include the knowledge and skills of infusion nurses. It is vital that they provide their assessments and input during the long-term management of MS.

REFERENCES

1. Namey M. *A Nursing Update: 2007*. Teaneck NJ: IOMSN Consensus Group. Teaneck, In press.

2. Decadron phosphate [package insert]. Whithouse Station, NJ: Merck & Co., 2001.

3. Methyprednisolone package insert.

4. Novantrone package insert.

5. Galetta SL, Markowitz C. US FDA-approved disease-modifying treatments for multiple sclerosis. Review of adverse effect profiles. *CNS Drugs*. 2005;19:1–14.

6. Cyclophosphamide Package Insert.

7. Goodin DS, Frohman EM, Garmany GP Jr, et al. Disease modifying therapies in multiple sclerosis: Report of the Therapeutics and Technology Assessment Subcommittee of the American Academy of Neurology and the MS Council for Clinical Practice Guidelines. *Neurology*. 2002;58:169–178.

8. Natalizumab Package Insert.

9. Yousry TA, Habil DM, Major EO, et al. Evaluation of patients treated with natalizumab for progressive multifocal leukoencephalopathy. *N Engl J Med*. 2006;354:924–933.

10. LaRocca NG. Psychosocial Issues in Multiple Sclerosis. In Halper J, Holland NJ, eds. *Comprehensive Nursing Care in Multiple Sclerosis*. New York: Demos V; 1997:83–107.

11. Fischer JS, Foley FW, Aiken JE, et al. What do we really know about cognitive dysfunction, affective disorders, and stress in multiple sclerosis? A practitioner's guide. *J Neuro Rehab*. 1994;8:151–164.

12. Goldman Consensus Group. The Goldman Consensus statement on depression in multiple sclerosis. *Multiple Sclerosis*. 2007;11:328–337.

CHAPTER 7

Promoting Adherence to Complex Protocols

Marie A. Namey

Multiple sclerosis (MS) is a complex disease that involves physical, psychological, and cognitive symptoms that affect adherence, particularly adherence to complex injectable protocols. Symptom management treatments have been available for many years for weakness, bowel and bladder disturbance, and other patient concerns. Many of these interventions are complicated for the patient to manage (medications, strategies to empty the bowel and bladder, issues of anxiety and depression). Since 1993, medications have been available that can affect the course of the disease. For the first time since MS was described, there is pharmacologic optimism. These treatment interventions are more complicated than previous treatments because they are injectable medications (see Chapter 4) that may or may not produce obvious change and benefit immediately.

Additionally, the provision of healthcare has changed dramatically in the past 20 to 25 years. Years ago, healthcare professionals made decisions for patients. Today healthcare providers are moving toward a sharing, caring, and more interactive partnership with the patient. Healthcare providers support two-way communication, and provide information to patients to allow them to make their own informed healthcare decisions. Finally, the complex health insurance system challenges both patients and healthcare providers with its own complexities.

The information presented in this chapter differentiates between the terms *compliance* and *adherence*, and reviews the theoretical perspectives related to the concepts of adherence and nonadherence.

The aim of this chapter is to focus on nursing strategies that promote adherence (primarily education, advocacy, and communication) and to foster the patient-related self-care regimens necessary when living with a chronic illness.

From Compliance to Adherence

The terms *compliance* and *adherence* have been used interchangeably in healthcare literature. Compliance is the extent to which the patient's behavior (in terms of taking medications, following diets, or executing other lifestyle changes) coincides with the clinical prescriptions (1). The core elements of compliance imply a power relationship assumed by the providers of care—the healthcare professionals—and exerted over the recipient—the patient. It also implies some coercion, domination, and possibly negotiation. Compliance is a one-way communication in which a message, in the form of a direction or order, is sent to a receiver. Also, negative authoritarian connotations are associated with the word *compliance*. If an outcome is positive, the healthcare professional has been successful; negative outcomes often are attributed to the patient. Compliance is not a good model in long-term chronic illness or disability.

From a nursing perspective, *adherence* is the preferred term, and can be defined as "the active, voluntary, and collaborative involvement of the patient in a mutually acceptable course of behavior that results in a desired preventative or therapeutic outcome" (2). The core elements include partnership, mutually established goals, and a therapeutic alliance. A considerable challenge for chronically ill individuals is adherence to prescribed medical regimens or planned lifestyle changes. Problems with following recommendations (both pharmacologic and nonpharmacologic) are well documented in the literature, with estimates of nonadherence between 30% and 70%, with an average of approximately 50% (3).

The prevalence of nonadherence has been reported extensively in the literature: Cardiac patients do not exercise, hemodialysis patients do not follow diets for fluid recommendations, and brain or spinal cord injury patients do not follow their treatment plans. Only one study has examined adherence to treatment in patients with MS. Mohr and coworkers (4) reported the correlation of inaccurate expectations of patients with MS who were started on interferon beta 1a (Betaseron) and the discontinuation of medication. Patients who were started on Betaseron and had overly optimistic expectations of functional improvement were at greater risk of discontinuing therapy than were those who had more realistic expectations.

Table 7-1 summarizes nursing strategies that can help to improve adherence.

TABLE 7-1
Nursing Strategies to Improve Adherence

Nurse–Patient Relationship
> Empathize with patient
> Establish a trusting relationship
> Be accessible
> Provide reassurance
> Help set realistic expectations
> Recognize the impact of treatment on lifestyle
> Maintain a sense of hope

Communication
> Discuss diagnosis and treatment options
> Discuss treatment plan selected
> Offer reinforcement
> Discuss timetable for follow-up

Education about Treatment
> Explain rationale for treatment
> Provide written information
> Provide simple, structured directions
> Arrange for additional support to help patient and family:
>> —Understand treatment plan
>> —Implement plan
>> —Integrate plan into current situation

Continuity of Care
> Provide indirect support (telephone, letters)
> Schedule regular follow-up
> Discuss adherence at each visit
> Use nonjudgmental approach to discussing adherence
> Facilitate access to health care system
> Facilitate access to home care agencies
> Refer to appropriate specialists (physical therapy, occupational therapy, social work, psychology)
> Encourage use of community resources
> Advocate for access to care

Theoretical Models Related to Adherence

Methods for dealing with adherence–nonadherence have been guided by several theoretical models in healthcare. These theoretical models offer some explanation or rationale from a variety of frameworks. The concept of adherence–nonadherence is influenced by a variety of factors. Haynes (1) identified more than 200 variables that have been examined in relation to adherence. No consistent relationship has been identified with age, gender, social class, marital status, or personality traits. More than 4,000 reports have been published on how to control nonadherence. Factors identified to affect adherence have been categorized as (a) patient variables, (b) disease variables, (c) treatment variables, (d) patient–healthcare provider relationship, and (e) clinical setting. Data also suggest that adherence can be enhanced in settings that provide continuity of care. The health belief model, social learning theory, self-efficacy model, transtheoretical model, and harm reduction model are all helpful in explaining patient behavior and behavior change. Each of these theories is explored in more detail and reviewed in terms of its relevance to the person with MS.

Health Belief Model

The health belief model reinforces the tenet that a patient's beliefs and expectations are important. In this model, adherence is enhanced by a patient's perception that his susceptibility to an illness is great or that he actually has the disease. A patient is also more likely to adhere to therapeutic regimens when he believes that the treatment will be effective, thus reducing its threat to him (5). Additionally, a patient weighs the advantages and disadvantages of participating in a behavior. Perceived risks, such as discomfort, monetary expense, and inconvenience, reduce the likelihood of patient adherence. Nonadherence is more common when a person doubts the safety of the regimen or is aware of untoward side effects.

Adherence rates are typically higher among patents with acute conditions as compared with those having chronic conditions (6).

Patients with MS frequently fall into one of two classifications: those who are proactive about disease management and those who are uninvolved or more passive about treatment. For example, once a person is given the diagnosis of MS and is aware that he may experience subsequent symptoms or exacerbations of the illness, he may choose to actively seek treatments for symptoms or use disease-modifying medications. A patient may be concerned about relieving symptoms now and preventing disability in the future. He may select a proactive approach to his illness and seek healthcare providers who are aggressive in treating MS. However, if a patient believes that MS will not negatively impact her life, he may choose to minimize his interactions with healthcare providers and not seek treatment. Or, if a person with MS thinks that treatments are too expensive or inconvenient, he may be hesitant to follow recommendations.

Social Learning Theory

Social learning theory is described as (a) a cognitive theory that examines what people think, and (b) how these thoughts influence their behavior. The social learning theory is also known as the *locus of control theory*. Relating this theory to health, patients may believe that their health is either under their control (internally controlled) or not under their control (externally controlled). The theory holds that there may be a reciprocal interaction between the individual and environmental influences on her behavior (6). A person with MS may not follow a prescribed regimen because of an underlying belief that her health status is beyond control and determined by outside forces. An individual with an internal locus of control belief may be more likely to follow a prescribed treatment regimen, because she believes that her behavior controls the outcome to some extent (7).

The healthcare provider should involve the MS patient in her own care. To help increase motivation and adherence, the patient should be involved in making decisions about care. The patient must be viewed as an active participant in the clinical decision-making process. She should be encouraged to express her concerns and expectations and allowed to participate in treatment decisions.

Self-Efficacy Theory

Self-efficacy is the belief that a person can or cannot perform a specific behavior. The self-efficacy model, as proposed by Bandura (8), considers the capability of a person performing a behavior that leads to outcomes. Self-efficacy is assessed by asking a patient whether he believes a particular behavior could be accomplished. Setting short-term goals, in combination with feedback about accomplishing these goals, can increase self-efficacy. For example, a person with MS may not believe that he is capable of giving an injection as a treatment for MS. Although he believes that there is benefit from an injectable medication, the patient may not be comfortable performing the procedure because he is not skilled in the technique and is uncomfortable with the idea of self-injection.

Another effective method to increase self-efficacy is modeling (9). Modeling uses patients who are successful in coping with certain problems to act as models for other patients. Group support sessions and group education can be an effective forum that allows group members to help each other solve problems.

Providing recent, factual information to the patient and providing educational materials in both verbal and written form (or through the use of videos or other multimedia) can enhance self-efficacy. Offering reassurance and encouraging self-care skills strengthens the likelihood of patient adherence.

Behavioral Change

Behavioral change is influenced by two models: the *transtheoretical model* and the *harm-reduction model*. The transtheoretical model accepts the fact that change is a long-term process, and behavioral change is a dynamic and individualized process. Change does not occur suddenly, and the person who is attempting to change goes through a series of ups and downs in the process of developing new habits. The major construct of the transtheoretical models is that change is incremental, not monumental (10).

The harm-reduction model supports the philosophy that the healthcare practitioner approaches the patient in a nonjudgmental manner and that individual rights are of prime importance. The healthcare provider works with the patient to meet personally established goals. Additionally, clients have the right to make personal decisions. And, obviously, the overall goal is to reduce harm. There are well-defined stages of behavioral change according to the harm reduction model, including:

1. *Precontemplation*: being aware of the problem but not yet planning to change
2. *Contemplative*: acknowledging a problem and thinking about solving it
3. *Preparation*: developing a plan for change
4. *Action*: progressing toward a goal with support
5. *Maintenance*: reaching and sustaining a goal
6. *Termination*: winning the struggle

No single study or theory has been able to offer a universally acceptable and effective solution to the problem of nonadherence. Understanding the influence of all factors is important.

The Nurse's Role in Promoting Adherence

Many factors affect adherence. As the largest segment of healthcare providers, nurses are in a primary position to enhance patient care, impact healthcare delivery, and play a major role in promoting adherence. A total systems approach (including cognitive, emotional, and behavioral variables) affects adherence, not any one single factor. Adherence to prescribed regimens is a problem-prone aspect of care. Nurses providing care to patients with a chronic illness are faced with many challenges. Nurses are advocates for all health-impaired individuals, and are concerned about the behaviors of the healthcare population. Nursing is a human service that relies on providing information so that the individual receiving care can make informed decisions. Historically, healthcare providers have negatively affected patients by excluding them from conversations about their care. Allowing patients to participate in discussions about treatment and care is paramount to adherence (11).

The major factors that positively affect adherence are:

+ Patient knowledge and understanding
+ Communication between patient and healthcare provider

+ Quality of interaction between patient and healthcare provider and patient satisfaction
+ Social support involving family system
+ Health beliefs and attitudes
+ Factors associated with the illness

Certainly, other factors positively affect adherence, and each nurse brings to the patient interaction attributes that affect adherence.

Strategies to Improve Adherence

The unpredictable course of MS may cause patients to view their disease as uncontrollable, leading to less self-efficacy and expectations about its management. Although MS is not a curable disease, treatments can be clearly outlined. The treatment regimen should be clearly stated by the practitioner. The timing of the message and the clarity of its organization can have powerful effects on reception, comprehension, and retention, which are key elements to adherence.

For example, following a general education session about MS, a patient (and family) should be made aware of treatment options for symptom management as well as treatment options for disease-modifying therapy. In many cases, patients may not be aware of the variety of treatments available for MS symptoms and disease. They may be overwhelmed with a sense of defeat on hearing the diagnosis of MS. Patient education should be aimed at strengthening self-efficacy expectations. Including the patient and family in the discussion of treatment options and the treatment plan selected can help enhance adherence. Educational information should be clear and unambiguous and written in easy-to-read print. Nontechnical language should be used. The language, pacing, and style used by the healthcare practitioner have an impact on patient understanding. Increasing the patient's knowledge of medication or disease does not affect adherence unless he is taught how to implement it in the treatment regimen (9). Nurses must emphasize that even the most effective drug protocols have limited benefit if patients don't adhere to the treatment regimens.

Taal and coworkers (12) found that patient education can be effective in changing knowledge, behaviors, and health status for patients with rheumatoid arthritis. Patients with MS, another chronic illness, may benefit similarly from education that positively affects adherence. Patient education can help patients to make decisions about their treatment regimens. Hogue (13) reported that nurses generally take more time to educate patients than do physicians. Nurses also are more likely to pay attention to their patients' social situation, which could affect treatment and adherence. A positive, hopeful attitude presented by the nurse may also improve adherence. In this author's experience, this has held true during the past decade and more. This conclusion has also been embraced by the pharmaceutical manufacturers of injectable medications, which provide patients with access to nurses who provide ongoing assistance to patients and families through education and support.

Relationship with Healthcare Provider

The relationship between the healthcare provider and the patient is of extreme importance in providing care for an individual with a chronic illness. Nurses who specialize in the care of individuals with MS validate patient experiences. Nurses can be instrumental in empowering patients with a chronic illness, such as MS. They can help patients and their families make informed decisions by sharing their experiences and expertise and by supporting the patient's priorities and decisions in a nonthreatening way. Developing a timetable for follow-up and planning regular follow-up strengthens adherence.

Social Support Network

The experience of MS affects not only the person with the disease but also family and friends. Including family members and promoting their involvement in MS care is of paramount importance. Care partners should be included in all education and follow-up appointments. If a person with MS is started on an injectable therapy, the physical and emotional support of family members is essential. However, family support sometimes is not enough, and patients need to extend their support network to include others.

Contacts with church groups can fulfill both emotional and spiritual needs. Community and peer support can be invaluable. The resources of the National Multiple Sclerosis Society have been available to individuals with MS for the past 60 years.

Health Beliefs and Attitudes

Health beliefs, attitudes, and patient expectations all affect adherence. Helping the patient and family to determine realistic expectations is a nursing strategy that promotes adherence. If a patient has unrealistic expectations of what a particular medication or treatment recommendation can do, she may be less likely to continue the treatment. In the case of MS, the treatment goal is basically to maintain—rather than improve—function. The goal of the injectable medications (Avonex, Betaseron, Copaxone, and Rebif) is to provide protection from frequent, severe exacerbations. The immunomodulatory medications have been proven to reduce the frequency and severity of exacerbations. All four agents (Avonex®, Betaseron®, Copaxone®, and Rebif®) have also been shown to decrease the lesion accrual seen on magnetic resonance imaging.

However, some individuals may start an injectable neuroimmunomodulatory medication with the hope that their symptoms will improve or dissipate.

Other factors associated with MS, including physical impairments, emotional distress, and cognitive deficits, can impact adherence. Visual disturbances can interfere with a patient's ability to read instructions and to prepare and take medications. Mobility problems, such as tremor, fatigue, and weakness, can prevent the patient from accessing clinical services, including rehabilitation.

Uncertainty about the future course of the disease, irrational fears, anxiety, and a sense of feeling out of control are common problems faced by patients with MS.

Emotional distress or underlying psychiatric illness can interfere with a patient's ability and interest in following medical recommendations. For example, an individual who is depressed may not be motivated to continue physical therapy exercises.

In addition, approximately 50% of people with MS experience some degree of cognitive impairment. Difficulty with learning and recalling new material may present problems in remembering to take medications or follow treatment regimens. Carrying out multistep procedures, such as self-injection or self-catheterization, may be difficult or impossible.

Related financial concerns may affect patients' adherence to following expensive treatment regimens. And, of course, cultural variables play a role in adherence to treatment management protocols.

Other factors that negatively influence adherence are the complexity of advice, a poor relationship between healthcare provider and patient, and the interference of advice with personal beliefs, goals, and expectations (14).

Summary

Multiple sclerosis is a complex disease, and adherence is a complex and dynamic concept, particularly for those providing nursing interventions to patients with chronic illness.

A wide range of factors affect adherence in both positive and negative ways. With the development of new, effective treatments for MS that are somewhat complicated, education of the patient and family is essential. Communication and accessibility of the healthcare provider are also key elements to promote adherence. The author is optimistic that the role of the nurse in providing care to individuals with a chronic illness, particularly MS, is a catalyst for adherence.

REFERENCES

1. Haynes RB, Taylor DW, Sackett DL. *Compliance in Healthcare*. Baltimore: John Hopkins University Press; 1979:1.

2. Multiple sclerosis: Key issues in nursing management. *Medicalliance*. 1998:5–11.

3. Anderson RJ, Kirk LM. Methods of improving patient compliance in chronic disease states. *Arch Intern Med*. 1982;142:1673–1675.

4. Mohr DC, Goodkin DE, Likosky W, et al. Therapeutic expectations of patients with multiple sclerosis upon initiating interferon-beta-1b: Relationship to adherence to treatment. *Multiple Sclerosis*. 1996;2:222–226.

5. Becker MH. The health belief model in personal health behavior. *Health Educ Monograph*. 1974;2:324–473.

6. Osterberg L, Blasche T. Adherence to medication. *N Engl J Med*. 2005;35:5:487–497.

7. Rotter JB. Generalized expectancies for internal versus external control of reinforcement. *Psychol Monogr*. 1966;80(1):1–28.

8. Bandura A. Self-efficacy: Toward a unifying theory of behavioral change. *Psychol Rev*. 1977;84:191–215.

9. Bandura A. *Social Learning Theory*. New York: General Learning Press, 1971.

10. Bradley-Springer L. Patient education for behavior change: Help from the transtheoretical and harm reduction models. *JANC*. 1996;7(Suppl 1):23–34.

11. Boczkowski JA, Zeichner A, DeSanto N. Neuroleptic compliance among chronic schizophrenic outpatients: An intervention outcome report. *J Consult Clin Psychol*. 1985; 53:666–671.

12. Taal E, Rasker JJ, Seydel ER, Wiegman O. Health status, adherence with health recommendations, self-efficacy and social support in patients with rheumatoid arthritis. *Patient Educ Counsel*. 1993;20:63–76.

13. Hogue CC. Nursing and Compliance. In: Haynes RB, Taylor DW, Sackett DL, eds. *Compliance in Healthcare*. Baltimore: Johns Hopkins University Press, 1979.

14. DiMatteo MR, DiNicola DD. *Achieving Patient Compliance: The Psychology of the Medical Practitioner's Role*. New York: Pergamon Press, 1982.

CHAPTER 8

The Role of Research in Nursing Practice

Elsie E. Gulick

Standards of practice for nursing, as promulgated by the American Nursing Association, explicitly state that nurses should use research findings in practice to improve healthcare outcomes and participate in the research process to discover, examine, and test knowledge, theories, and creative approaches to practice (1). Clinical nursing research is designed to generate knowledge to guide nursing practice and to improve the health and quality of life of patients (2). This chapter briefly discusses the purpose and value of research in clinical nursing practice, followed by a more detailed discussion regarding the involvement of nurses in the utilization and participation in research to effect best evidence-based practice (EBP).

A discipline is characterized by a body of knowledge that represents a unique perspective (3). Nursing is a practice discipline charged to treat human responses to both potential and actual health problems (4). Although nurses use knowledge developed by both academic and professional disciplines in this situation, knowledge from the perspective of nursing is essential for the implementation of humanistic and holistic nursing care (5).

Knowledge held to be of value in the discipline of nursing includes that obtained from research, as well as from aesthetics, ethics, and personal sources (6). Knowledge from empirical research emerges from descriptive, explanatory, or predictive methods of research; aesthetic knowledge is gained through

perceiving and empathizing the uniqueness of clients; ethical and moral knowledge reflect philosophic views regarding what is good or right behavior; and
personal knowledge emerges from an understanding of self and others. Both
quantitative and qualitative research can inform EBP (7).

Purpose and Value of Nursing Research

Nursing research is the conduct of systematic studies to generate new knowledge
or confirm existing knowledge through quantitative and qualitative methods (8).
Quantitative methods use deductive reasoning to systematically gather empirical
evidence about a specific research question or hypothesis (2). This method uses
evidence that is analyzed with statistical procedures to yield answers to the
research question or hypothesis. Qualitative research uses inductive methods that
employ naturalistic investigations that place a heavy emphasis on understanding
the human experience as it is lived through careful collection and analysis of
subjective narratives (2). Qualitative research provides rich informative data that
was previously inaccessible and frequently helps investigators identify important
side issues related to the main research question (9). To be of value to nurses in
caring for patients, nursing research must be meaningful in terms of providing
knowledge to guide them in promoting health, preventing illness, or increasing
the potential for recovery from illness (10).

Escalating healthcare costs, downsizing in healthcare facilities and programs,
new treatment modalities and technologies, and demand by patients for quality
care are all indicators suggesting the need to change traditional forms of healthcare services. The impact that these complex indicators have on the outcomes of
healthcare must be evaluated through carefully designed research. Results from
carefully designed research benefit patients, nurses, healthcare agencies, and the
discipline of nursing.

Patients benefit from the utilization of nursing research in terms of enhanced
quality of patient care (11–18), reduced costs of services (15,17), and increased
satisfaction with care (19). As noted by Grady (20), nursing research findings have
enhanced the health and well-being of diverse populations in patient-focused and
holistic ways.

Nursing staff benefit by using research findings to improve nursing practice
and through actual participation in the research process. The utilization of
research findings by nurses to improve nursing practice enhances job satisfaction
and professionalism among the staff (11,17,18) as well as feelings of empowerment
(16,21). Increased job satisfaction among nursing staff benefits healthcare
organizations as a result of the increased likelihood of enhanced recruitment
and retention of nurses (22).

The discipline of nursing is enhanced through research by increasing the
scientific knowledge base underlying nursing practice. Donaldson (5) stated

"the knowledge of the discipline must ultimately support service to clients and the health of society." Furthermore, knowledge derived from nursing research, together with that of medical and other sciences, is essential for establishing meaningful healthcare policy change.

Research Involvement of Nursing Staff

All levels of nursing staff can and should participate in the research process, as stated in the nursing practice standards promulgated by the American Nurses Association (1).

Staff nurses are involved in various aspects of research utilization and/or in the actual conduct of research. First, all nurses must have a conceptual awareness of state-of-the-art research in their specialty practice area, even if some of the research findings are not currently adopted as part of their patient care interventions. Maintaining currency in state-of-the-art knowledge in one's practice area occurs by regular reading of research and clinical journals, surfing the Internet for relevant research, participating in nursing research committee activities within an organization, attendance at clinical research conferences, and active participation in professional organizations in nursing as well as in organizations that focus on specific diseases related to one's work. In addition to a conceptual awareness of current research findings, staff nurses need to use relevant clinical research to promote best EBP.

Involving staff nurses in clinical research aimed at promoting EBP is best accomplished using a team approach. Suggested composition of the team includes nurses involved in direct patient care, management, and research. Each team member has specific expertise that, when put together, creates a mechanism capable of facilitating best EBP.

Research Utilization for Promoting Evidence-Based Practice

Research utilization is the process of transforming research knowledge into practice (23). Evidence-based practice is the process of integrating clinical knowledge, judgment, and proficiency skills with the best available clinical evidence, such as nursing research, into patient care (24). A number of phases and steps are required in considering, planning, implementing, and evaluating the EBP process. The EBP process steps are numbered in the discussion that follows and correspond to the numbered boxes appearing in Figure 8-1.

The *Problem/Question Identification phase* begins with a consensus of a problem or unsolved question by nursing staff from ongoing interactions with

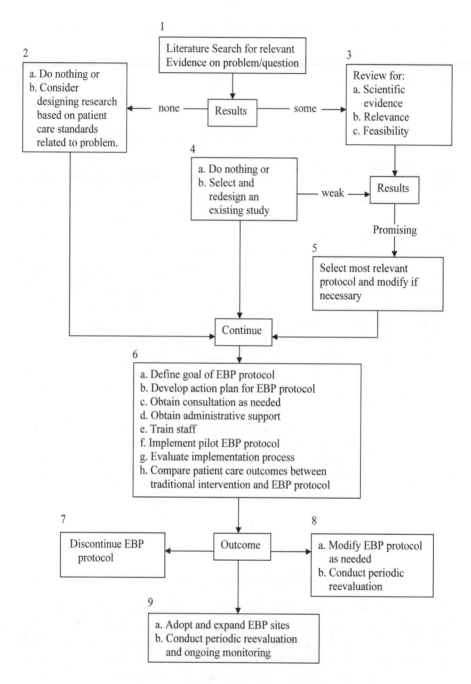

FIGURE 8-1.

Action steps used to determine whether an EBP change is warranted.

patients. Titler and colleagues (16,25) cite a number of problem- and knowledge-focused triggers that serve as catalysts for engaging in EBP to promote quality care. Problem-focused triggers include risk management data, process improvement data, internal/external benchmarking data, financial data, and identification of clinical problems. Knowledge-focused triggers include new research or other literature, national agencies or organizational standards and guidelines, philosophies of care, and questions from the Institutional Standards Committee. An individual or team of individuals begins the process by considering what environmental factors, such as prioritized goals of the organization, may have on the EBP protocol. This phase includes a search of literature pertaining to the proposed problem or unsolved question (step 1).

Resources for conducting literature searches include health databases accessible through the Internet. The Cumulative Index to Nursing and Allied Health Literature (CINAHL) is an online searchable index of primarily nursing information. The CANCERLIT database, developed by the U. S. National Cancer Institute, contains pertinent information on cancer. MEDLINE/PubMed is a U. S. government database provided free to the public; it encompasses medicine, nursing, dentistry, veterinary medicine, healthcare system, and preclinical sciences. The PsycINFO database is a compilation of psychology related information including medical, nursing, and education disciplines. The Cochrane Library, accessed at http://www.Cochrane.org/, features summary reviews of the literature. These reviews are conducted by experts and overseen by a quality assurance panel. The Agency for Healthcare Quality Research (AHRQ) is a federal agency that supports the development of evidence reports. The AHRQ is accessed at http://www.ahcpr.gov/; the dissemination of evidence-based guidelines through the agency's National Guideline Clearinghouse can be accessed at http://www.guideline.gov/. Techniques to improve database searching are described by Schoolmeesters (26), and published in an Internet guide for nurses. Both primary studies and research reviews should be examined for relevance to the EBP problem under consideration.

Primary studies are those published in the clinical literature. These include clinical trials, surveys, retrospective studies, and case reports (27). Research reviews critically summarize past research on a specific topic to draw conclusions that may inform research, practice, and policy (28). Research reviews include integrative reviews (review of methods, theories, and empirical results); meta-analysis (use of statistical methods to determine the overall effectiveness of a number of studies), systematic reviews (summarized evidence of a specific clinical problem using quantitative and qualitative research), and meta-summary reviews (summaries of processes or experiences of individuals using qualitative research) (28). Searching multiple sources of the literature will best inform the team of available evidence for their selected problem or question. When no studies of sufficient evidence are located, the team has two options: to do nothing to change the current problem (step 2a), or to consider designing a EBP protocol based on patient care standards related to the problem (step 2b).

The *Literature Summary phase* entails a critical review and summarization of articles pertaining to the EBP protocol (step 3a). Systematic and rigorous reviews for obtaining evidence in nursing research are essential in the planning phase of EBP, to enhance methodological rigor and subsequently the application of findings to practice (28). Evidence provided from the literature review should be rated for quality, quantity, and consistency (29). Quality evidence represents the aggregate of quality ratings for individual studies; quantity evidence represents the number of studies, sample size or power, and magnitude of intervention effect; and consistency evidence represents the extent to which similar findings are reported using similar and different designs for a specific topic. The AHRQ (29) lists important domains and elements in rating the quality of studies. Key domains and elements for observation studies include comparability of subjects, exposure or intervention, outcome measurements, and statistical analysis. Key domains and elements for systematic reviews include comparability of subjects, exposure or intervention, outcome measurement, and statistical analysis of data. Key domains and elements for randomized clinical trials include the study population, randomization, blinding, interventions, outcomes, and statistical analysis. All studies should identify the source of funding or sponsorship. The strength of reviewed evidence from the studies, in descending order of importance, are meta-analysis studies, individual experimental studies, quasi-experimental studies, nonexperimental studies (correlation, descriptive, or qualitative), case report or program evaluation, and opinion of respected authorities based on clinical experience.

The *Evidence Synthesis phase* requires a synthesis of evidence from the study findings and a determination of relevance and feasibility (risk, resources, readiness) for adopting, adapting, or ceasing further consideration of the proposed EBP protocol (step 3b,c). Results of the review of studies may lead to the conclusion that they either lack sufficient evidence, relevance, or feasibility. This may direct the team to consider doing nothing (step 4a) or to select and redesign an existing study (step 4b). Alternatively, the review that provides promising evidence may guide the team in selecting the most relevant EBP protocol and modify it slightly, if necessary (step 5). If the decision is to adopt with or without needed adaptations, EBP guidelines must be designed, and approvals from the organizational hierarchy must be sought. Additionally, specific outcomes must be identified and measures selected that are sensitive to detecting change as a result of adopting the proposed protocol. Outcome measures may include qualitative self-report techniques, quantitative self-report instruments, observational data, bio-physiologic data, and benchmarking data. Consideration must be given to the potential influence of patient characteristics (e.g., age, gender, level of education, ethnicity), patient's clinical condition, and nursing unit characteristics (e.g., skill mix, bed capacity, type of unit) on the outcome data (31). Sources for outcome measures are presented in Table 8-1.

The *Pilot phase* begins when the decision is to move forward with the implementation of the EBP protocol, and approval from the administration hierarchy

TABLE 8-1
Sources of Instruments for Measuring Outcomes

Source (Reference)	Description of Measures
Instruments for Clinical HealthCare Research, 3rd ed. (30)	Major areas of measurement include function, cognitive status, quality of life, social support, coping, hope, spirituality, sexuality, dietary intake, sleep, anxiety, depression, self-care activities, bowel elimination, cardiac parameters, dyspnea, fatigue, pain, skin integrity, mobility.
Measurement of Nursing Outcomes: Measuring Nursing Performance in Practice, Education, and Research, Vol. 1, 2nd ed. (32)	Provides validated measures that focus on clinical decision-making and performance in education, practice, and research. A copy of the scale is included in most cases.
Measurement of Nursing Outcomes: Client Outcomes and Quality of Care, Vol. 2, 2nd ed. (33)	Provides validated measures that focus on patient phenomena important to nursing practice, e.g. patient's functional status, distress, fear, empathy, satisfaction with care, and others. Evidence of validity and reliability are given and a copy of each scale.
Measurement of Nursing Outcomes: Self-Care and Coping, Vol. 3, 2nd ed. (34)	Provides validated measures that focus on client care, social support, quality of life, self-esteem, coping, and health promoting behaviors.
Nursing Quality Indicators: Measurement Instruments (35)	Contains nursing-sensitive measures for nonacute healthcare settings. Measures include indicators of pain management, ADL and IADL functioning, psychosocial interaction. Description, validity, sensitivity, and interpretability for the measures are presented.
Handbook of Neurologic Rating Scales (36)	Contains a chapter on scales used for MS patients that focus on disability level, upper and lower extremity functioning, cognitive functioning, quality of life, and fatigue. Validity estimates as well as advantages and disadvantages of the scale are presented.

has been granted (step 6a–d). This phase includes training staff and conducting a pilot study for the purpose of evaluating the process, guidelines, and outcomes pertaining to the EBP protocol (step 6e–h). Evaluation of the pilot study must include the process steps used to implement the EBP protocol as well as patient care outcomes. Evaluation of the process steps used for implementation of the EBP protocol is essential because the expected outcomes may not occur if the process is not carried out as intended. A comparison of patient care outcomes based on the traditional intervention with that of the EBP protocol is essential. If the desired evidence is not forthcoming from the pilot data, and revision is not considered appropriate, the EBP protocol may be discontinued (step 7). Based on the pilot evaluation, refinements of the protocol, if necessary, should be undertaken (step 8a,b).

The *Integration and Monitoring phase* involves instituting the revised or accepted EBP protocol in the desired nursing units. This must be done with continuing monitoring and analysis of the structure, process, and outcome data obtained from the environment, staff, patient and family, and cost/benefit data (step 9). Results of the EBP process and outcomes should be disseminated to other nurses through research/clinical practice conferences and publication.

Summary

Providing the best possible nursing care for patients requires nurses to utilize nursing research findings pertaining to their particular area of nursing practice. Together with best clinical judgment and existing professional skills, these research findings must have sufficient evidence to warrant adoption in their healthcare setting. Evidence-based practice guided by relevant research should enhance best practice and eliminate those practices that do not contribute to improved outcomes.

REFERENCES

1.   ANA. *Nursing: Scope & Standards of Practice*. American Nurses Association: Washington, DC, 2004.

2.   Polit DF, Beck CT. *Nursing Research: Principles and Methods*, 7th ed., Philadelphia: Lippincott Williams & Wilkins, 2004.

3.   Donaldson SK, Crowley DM. The discipline of nursing. *Nurs Outlook*. 1978;26:113–120.

4.   ANA. *Nursing: A Social Policy Statement*. Kansas City, MO: American Nurses Association, 1980.

5.   Donaldson SK. Nursing science for nursing practice. In: Omery A. Kasper CE, Page GG, eds. *In Search of Nursing Science*. Thousand Oaks, CA: Sage Publications; 1995:3–12.

6.   Carper BA. Fundamental patterns of knowing in nursing. *Adv Nur Sci*. 1978;1(1):13–23.

7.   Upshur REG. The status of qualitative research as evidence. In: Morse JM, Swanson JM, Kuzel AJ, eds. *The Nature of Qualitative Evidence*. Thousand Oaks, CA: Sage Publications; 2001:5–26.

8.   Blegen MA, Tripp-Reimer T. Nursing theory, nursing research, and nursing practice: Connected or separate? In: Dochterman JM, Grace HK , eds. *Current Issues in Nursing*, 6th ed. St. Louis: Mosby; 2001:44–51.

9.   Olson K. Using qualitative research in clinical practice In: Morse JM, Swanson JM, Kuzel AJ, eds. *The Nature of Qualitative Evidence*. Thousand Oaks, CA: Sage Publications; 2001:259–273.

10. Weiss SJ. Contemporary empiricism. In: Omery A, Kasper CE, Page GG, eds. *In Search of Nursing Science.* Thousand Oaks, CA: Sage Publications; 1995:13–26.

11. Happell B, Martin T. Exploring the impact of the implementation of a nursing clinical development unit program: What outcomes are evident? *Int J Mental Health Nurs.* 2004;13:177–184.

12. Haycock, C, Laser C, Keuth J, et al. Implementing evidence-based practice findings to decrease postoperative sternal wound infections following open heart surgery. *J Cardiovasc Nurs.* 2005;20(5):299–305.

13. Miranda MB, Gorski LA, LeFevre JG, et al. An evidence-based approach to improving care of patients with heart failure across the continuum. *J Nurs Care Qual.* 2002;17(1):1–14.

14. Christie W, Moore C. The impact of humor on patients with cancer. *Clin J Oncol Nurs.* 2005;9(2):211–218, 225–227.

15. Specht JP, Bergquist S, Frantz FA. Adoption of a research-based practice for treatment of pressure ulcers. *Nurs Clin North Am.* 1995;30(3):553–563.

16. Titler MG, Kleiber C, Steelman V, et al. Infusing research into practice to promote quality care. *Nurs Res.* 1994;43(5):307–313.

17. Sturkey EN, Linker S, Comeau E. Improving wound care outcomes in the home setting. *J Nurs Care Qual.* 2005;20(4):349–355.

18. Fink F, Thompson CJ, Bonnes D. Overcoming barriers and promoting the use of research in practice. *J Nurs Adm.* 2005;35(3):121–129.

19. Vega-Stromberg T, Holmes SB, Gorski L, Johnson BP. Road to excellence in pain management: Research, outcomes and direction (ROAD). *Jour Nurs Care Qual.* 2002;17(1):15–29.

20. Grady PA. Bringing research to life. *Appl Nurs Res.* 1998;11(1):1.

21. Cullen L, Greiner J, Greiner J, et al. Excellence in evidence-based practice: Organizational and unit exemplars. *Crit Care Nurs Clin N Am.* 2005;17:127–142.

22. Smeltzer CH, Hinshaw AS. Research: Clinical integration for excellent patient care. *Nurs Manag.* 1988;19(1):38–44.

23. Stetler CB. Updating the Stetler model of research utilization to facilitate evidence-based practice. *Nurs Outlook.* 2001;49(6):272–279.

24. Couvillon JS. How to promote or implement evidenced-based practice in a clinical setting. *Home Healthcare Manag Practice.* 2005;17(4):269–272.

25. Titler MG, Kleiber C, Steelman VJ, et al. The Iowa model of evidence-based practice to promote quality care. *Crit Care Nurs Clin N Amer.* 2001;13(4):497–509.

26. Schoolmeesters LJ. Techniques to improve database searching. In Fitzpatrick JJ, Montgomery KS, eds. *Internet for Nursing Research: A Guide to Strategies, Skills, and Resources.* New York: Springer Publishing Company; 2004:9–18.

27. Wysocki AB, Bookbinder M. Implementing clinical practice changes: A practical approach. *Home Healthcare Manag& Practice.* 2005;17(3):164–174.

28. Whittemore R. Combining evidence in nursing research: Methods and implications. *Nurs Res.* 2005;54(1):67–62.

29. Agency for Healthcare Research and Quality. Systems to rate the strength of scientific evidence. Retrieved from http://www.ahcpr.gov/clinic/epcsums/strengthsum.htm Jan 23 2006.

30. Frank-Stromborg M, Olsen SJ. *Instruments for Clinical Health-Care Research,* 3rd ed. Sudbury, MA: Jones and Bartlett Publishers, 2004.

31. Titler MG. Outcomes Management for quality improvement. In: Dochterman JM, Grace HK, eds. *Current Issues in Nursing,* 6th ed. St. Louis: Mosby; 2001:246–254.

32. Waltz CF, Jenkins LS. *Measurement of Nursing Outcomes: Measuring Nursing Performance in Practice, Education, and Research,* Vol. 1, 2nd ed. New York: Springer Publishing Company, 2001.

33. Strickland OL, DiIorio C. *Measurement of Nursing Outcomes: Client Outcomes and Quality of Care,* Vol. 2, 2nd ed. New York: Springer Publishing Company, 2003.

34. Strickland OL, DiIorio C. *Measurement of Nursing Outcomes: Self Care and Coping,* Vol. 3, 2nd ed. New York: Springer Publishing Company, 2003.

35. ANA. *Nursing Quality Indicators beyond Acute Care: Measurement Instruments.* Washington, D.C.: American Nurses Association, 2000.

36. Herndon R, Greenstein JI. Multiple sclerosis and demyelinating diseases. In: Herndon RM, ed. *Handbook of Neurologic Rating Scales,* 2nd ed. New York: Demos; 2006:169–193.

CHAPTER 9

Research Coordinator: Another Dimension of Multiple Sclerosis Nursing

Linda A. Morgante

We are in an exciting and hopeful time in the field of multiple sclerosis (MS) treatment. Successful clinical trials have given us six treatments that alter the natural history of the disease. Interferon beta-1b (Betaseron), interferon beta-1a (Avonex), interferon beta-1a (Rebif), and glatiramer acetate (Copaxone) are commercially available in the United States, Canada, and parts of Europe. Mitoxantrone (Novantrone) demonstrated a positive effect on worsening MS and was approved in the United States. Recently, natalizumab (Tysabri) was also added to the arsenal of treatment options. Several regimens to relieve symptoms are also available because of positive effects measured in clinical trials (e.g., modafinil, Provigil). Many other drug trials currently in progress or being proposed will help continue to make a difference in the lives of people with MS.

The nursing profession lends itself to the work of coordinating clinical trials because the task involves caring for patients and families, moving systematically through a complicated process, communicating with a variety of professionals, being highly organized, and knowing how to prioritize. Good nursing care is the key to keeping patients healthy and safe during the time in which they participate in a trial. Nurses utilize clinical, interpersonal, administrative, and creative skills to help patients emerge triumphant through the rigors of a clinical trial.

This chapter focuses on the responsibilities of the nurse coordinating a clinical trial in MS. It includes information regarding informed consent, the role of the Institutional Review Board (IRB), adverse event reporting, audits, patient recruitment and selection, patient retention, the concepts of hope versus false hope, and nursing care issues specific to MS.

Overview of the Roles and Responsibilities of the Research Nurse Coordinator

The research nurse coordinator enjoys an ever-expanding role that includes educator, advocate, mediator, and recruiter. The nurse is responsible for over seeing everyday study tasks, such as managing data, ensuring adherence to the protocol, providing leadership, and helping the members of the research team to sustain their commitment to the protocol (1). With the variety of available treatments in MS, the nurse must also use ethics-based critical thinking skills when making decisions regarding whether a patient is appropriate to participate in a clinical trial.

The following question should be addressed when assessing the eligibility of each patient: Do the benefits outweigh the risks for this particular individual? The patient's safety and interests are of prime concern when looking at the risk–benefit ratio, and there are ethical principles that help provide a foundation for answering this question. Four of these principles are: *autonomy*, respecting the individual's right to self-determination; *justice*, fair balance for all; *beneficence*, doing what is right and good for the individual; and *veracity*, telling the truth. The consensus of the team regarding a patient's participation in a particular clinical trial will help to provide a variety of opinions and points of view, and it can help to ensure that the decision process follows an ethical pathway and results in a satisfactory outcome.

In addition to protecting human rights and ensuring patient safety, the research nurse coordinator is responsible for nurturing patient retention, maintaining regulatory files (Tables 9-1 and 9-2), providing accurate documentation, promoting adherence to the protocol, clarifying false expectations, recognizing and reporting adverse events, and inspiring hope.

The following sections will elaborate on many of these responsibilities.

TABLE 9-1
Study Files Notebook—What Is Included

1. Protocol—all versions
2. Protocol amendments
3. Consent forms—all versions
4. Investigator's brochure
5. 1572 forms and all updates
6. Curricula vitae of all those listed on the 1572
7. IRB approvals
8. IRB membership
9. IRB correspondence
10. Safety reports
11. SAE reports
12. Laboratory documents (normal values and certificates)
13. Drug accountability log
14. Sponsor correspondence
15. Monitoring log
16. Enrollment log

TABLE 9-2
Definition of Terms

1572 Form. The official document that secures the investigator's commitment to conduct the trial in accordance with FDA guidelines.

Case report forms. Concise information reflective of the source documents entered into duplicating forms that are collected and returned to the sponsor for data entry.

Investigator's brochure. A detailed, confidential description of the structure and formulation of the investigational drug, a summary of all the studies conducted using the product, and a review of adverse events associated with the drug (3).

Protocol. A framework for the conduct of the study that includes detailed, confidential information regarding the study's objectives, background, rationale, inclusion and exclusion criteria, designs, methods for data collection and entry, adverse event reporting, randomization, and end points.

Source documents. Documents that contain all the original clinical information gathered during a visit, which can be entered into a worksheet or detailed in the medical record.

TABLE 9-3
Ethical Milestones

The Nuremberg Code, 1947. Established the guidelines for informed consent, including provisions for withdrawal from studies, protection against suffering or injuries, and the inclusion of a risk–benefit rationale.
The Declaration of Helsinki, 1964. Expanded the principles established in the Nuremberg Code to further ensure the safety of human subjects by broadening the concept of informed consent. Also focused on investigator integrity and experience in conducting clinical trials.
The Belmont Report. Cornerstone statement of ethical principles upon which the federal regulations for the protection of subjects are based. It includes three basic principles: respect for individuals (captured in the informed consent), beneficence (captured in the risk–benefit assessment), and justice (captured in the selection of research subjects).
FDA Regulations, 1981. Directly derived from the ethical principles described in the Belmont Report; oversees all the ethical aspects of clinical trial work.

Protecting Human Rights: A Historical Perspective

History is one of our best teachers. A review of the historical events that have influenced the formation of the laws regulating the conduct of clinical research provides an important foundation for nurses who coordinate research studies (Table 9-3). These historical highlights paved the way for the ethical standards that guide clinical trials and ensure a participant's autonomy and right to self-determination. In addition to establishing standards, specific trial designs (Table 9-4) and levels of study or trial phases (Table 9-5) were developed as models for clinical study. The three most notable events are: The Nuremberg Doctors Trial (1946), the Thalidomide Tragedy (1960s), and the Tuskegee Syphilis Study (1972) (2).

The Nuremberg Doctors Trial

During World War II, the U.S. government funded studies concerning issues related to the "effectiveness of the war effort—dysentery, influenza, malaria, wounds, venereal disease, and physical hardships" (3). The subjects were uninformed prisoners, people institutionalized in homes for the mentally retarded or in psychiatric facilities, and our own military personnel. At the same time, the Nazi concentration camps became the setting for outrageous human experimentation (3).

The Nuremberg Trials that followed the war exposed and convicted those Nazis responsible for the atrocities in the camps and established a code to protect human subjects. The Nuremberg Code, drafted in 1947, established the basic guidelines for informed consent, including provisions for withdrawal, protection against suffering or injuries, and the inclusion of a risk–benefit rationale (2).

TABLE 9-4
Trial Designs

Open label. The investigators and patients are aware of what drug or device is being tested.
Single-blinded study. The patient is blinded to the treatment, but the investigator is aware of whatever is being tested.
Double-blinded study. Neither the investigator nor the patient is aware of who has been randomly (by chance) assigned the treatment or the placebo. This is a common design, providing the most reliable and scientific data, and involving a large sample size. It is often conducted at multiple study sites.
Cross-over study. Participants receive either placebo or commercial therapy for a specific time, then investigational drug for the remainder. This type is usually double-blind, randomized, and allows for periods during which treatment is not given ("wash out") so as not to blur data from one phase to another.

TABLE 9-5
Trial Phases

Phase I. Designed to determine the metabolism and pharmacologic actions of a drug on human subjects. This phase helps to determine the side effects associated with increasing doses of the drug, and helps to gain early evidence on the drug's effectiveness. Approximately 20 to 80 subjects are enrolled, and the trial is of a short duration.
Phase II. Well-controlled, closely monitored studies to evaluate the effectiveness of a drug for a particular indication. Subjects are people with the disease. This phase helps to determine the short-term side effects and risks of the drug. Several hundred subjects are usually enrolled. In MS care, Phase II studies often involve MRI findings.
Phase III. Expanded trials performed after preliminary evidence suggests drug may be effective. This phase is intended to gather additional information regarding effectiveness and safety of the drug. It often includes several hundred to several thousand subjects, and introduces the Data Safety Monitoring Committee.
Phase IV. Post-marketing studies are needed to test an approved product on different groups; change labeling (i.e., modalities for storing drug); and look at different issues that concern customers (i.e., use of an autoinjector).

The Thalidomide Tragedy

Thalidomide was approved as a sedative in Europe during the late 1950s. Samples of the drug were distributed by the manufacturer to doctors in the United States in order to collect safety and efficacy data on pregnant women. Years later, it was discovered that thalidomide was extremely damaging to the fetus. The Senate subcommittee that followed, chaired by Hubert Humphrey, exposed the fact that the subjects were never informed that they were being given an experimental substance, nor had they been asked to give their consent. Another senate subcommittee chaired by Senator Estes Ketover looked into the business practices of pharmaceutical companies. The findings of these two committees led to the passage of the drug amendment to the Food, Drug, and Cosmetic Act, with language added to that bill requiring researchers to inform subjects of the drug's experimental nature and to receive their consent before starting the research (2).

The Tuskegee Syphilis Study

For nearly two decades, beginning in the early 1950s, the natural course of latent syphilis was studied in 400 African American men. Although penicillin was available to treat the disease 10 years into the study, the United States Department of Health decided to withhold treatment to achieve its goal. In 1972, the Associated Press uncovered the story and, as a reaction to the publicity, Congress held hearings on experimentation using human subjects. The study was terminated in 1972. In 1974, Congress passed the National Research Act, which created the National Commission for the Protection of Human Subjects, and wrote the Ethical Principles and Guidelines for the Protection of Human Subjects of Research (the Belmont Report). The Belmont Report included requirements for informed consent and review of research by Institutional Review Boards, and became the foundation for the U.S. Food and Drug Administration (FDA) regulations that govern the conduct of clinical trials.

Protecting Human Rights: The Institutional Review Board

The IRB is responsible for making a risk–benefit assessment of each clinical trial and ensuring that all projects both conform to institutional policies and meet local, state, and federal rules and regulations. The IRB also conducts annual reviews of ongoing research projects and makes appropriate recommendations.

The IRB makes a determination to approve a research project based on the following considerations (3):

+ Risks to subjects are minimized
+ Risks to subjects are reasonable in relation to anticipated benefits
+ Selection of subjects is equitable
+ Informed consent is obtained from the subjects or from the subjects' legally authorized representative
+ The research has a rational scientific basis, and the methodology has scientific validity
+ The research plan makes adequate provision for monitoring the data collected to ensure the safety of subjects
+ There are adequate provisions to protect the privacy of subjects and maintain the confidentiality of data

The study coordinator may be responsible for IRB submissions. To ensure approval of new projects, the entire protocol, a synopsis, and the informed consent must be submitted for review, often first by a subcommittee of experts in related fields. The IRB must be notified of any serious adverse events that occur during the trial, and periodically (usually annually) it undertakes a review of the status of the study. A new study coordinator may obtain permission to attend an IRB meeting to help obtain a sense of this arduous process.

Protecting Human Rights: Informed Consent

The concept of informed consent is based on the ethical principles of full disclosure and the right of self-determination (4). Participants must be provided with a consent form that can be easily understood by the lay person and includes the following elements (2):

+ A statement that the study involves research
+ An explanation of the purpose of the research, a description of the procedures to be followed, and identification of any procedures that are experimental
+ The expected duration of the subject's participation
+ A description of any reasonably foreseeable risks or discomforts to the subject, including, if women who are able to have children are included in the study, risks with respect to childbearing or to a fetus
+ A description of any benefits to the subject that may be reasonably expected from the research
+ A disclosure of appropriate alternative procedures or courses of treatment, if any, that might be advantageous to the subject
+ A statement describing the extent to which confidentiality of records identifying the subject will be mentioned and, for FDA-supported research, noting the possibility that the FDA may inspect the records
+ For research involving more than minimal risk, an explanation as to whether compensation and medical treatment are available
+ An explanation of who should be contacted for answers to pertinent questions about the research and research subject's rights
+ A statement that participation is voluntary, refusal to participate will not result in any penalty or loss of services to which the subject is otherwise entitled, and that the subject may withdraw at any time without penalty

Nurses play a key role in helping patients understand the elements of the informed consent protocol. The specific concerns related to MS patients include difficulty comprehending the language of the consent, exaggerated expectations about the trial, and trouble concentrating on the often lengthy document.

TABLE 9-6
Adverse Events—Definitions for Safety Reporting

Adverse drug experience. Any unfavorable and unintended sign (including an abnormal laboratory finding), symptom, or disease temporally associated with the use of a medicinal (investigational) product, whether related to the medicinal (investigational) product or not (9).
Serious adverse drug experience. Any experience that results in death, a life-threatening adverse event, inpatient hospitalization or prolongation of hospitalization, a persistent or significant disability or incapacity, or congenital anomaly (9).
Unexpected adverse drug experience. Any adverse experience, the specificity or severity of which is not consistent with the current investigator's brochure (9).

Educating and counseling patients and families regarding their rights during a trial and explaining the key elements in a clear concise manner help ensure that the consent process has been completed properly. If significant cognitive deficiencies are noted for a particular patient, a caregiver should be present to cosign the consent form. Documentation in the chart includes information regarding how the consent process was conducted, the date, and who witnessed the signature. It should also be noted that no study-related activities occurred before signing.

Reporting Serious Adverse Events

The research nurse coordinator is responsible for recognizing and reporting all adverse events in a trial (Table 9-6). The recording of any adverse event must be included in the source document and in the case report form and should describe the problem, the time started and resolved, and the etiology. Relationship to study drug and seriousness of the event must also be documented in both places. Figure 9-1 outlines the process for reporting adverse events in a clinical trial in the United States, and offers the research nurse a quick and accurate reference.

Recruitment and Patient Selection

Recruiting patients for trials in MS has become more difficult because of the commercial availability in the United States of six disease-modifying therapies: interferon beta 1–a (Avonex), interferon beta 1–a (Rebif), interferon beta-1b (Betaseron), glatiramer acetate (Copaxone), mitoxantrone (Novantrone), and natalizumab (Tysabri). Experimental therapies may be most attractive to patients who have not tolerated prior courses of treatment, have experienced

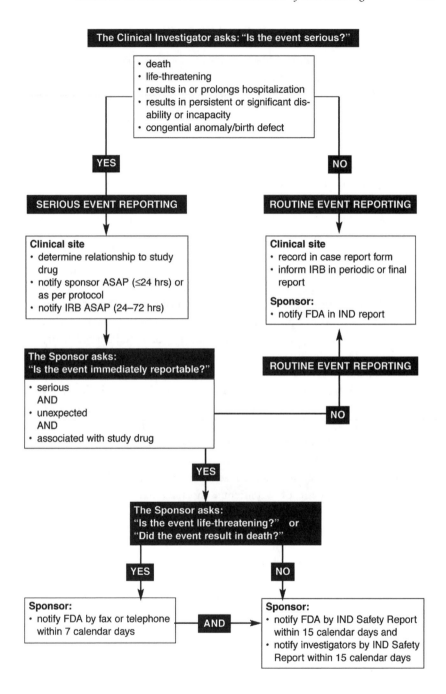

FIGURE 9-1

Reporting adverse drug events in the United States, immediately reportable (IR) and routine.
Reprinted with permission from *Research Nurse*, May/June 1998, p. 7.

disease worsening despite aggressive treatment, or wish to try an agent that is administered orally.

Steger (5) suggests that there are barriers and benefits to the recruitment process. These include "individual psychosocial factors, negative community attitudes, provider bias, restrictive inclusion/exclusion criteria, and research staff and site. Benefits for participation in studies include access to promising therapies, access to medical expertise, close medical attention, emotional support, and altruism" (5; p. 2).

Based on factors such as those cited by Steger, specific recruitment strategies can be developed. These include access to databases; review of patient files; retention of ongoing lists of eligible candidates; setting up of networks with local physicians (i.e., grand rounds); letters, phone calls, and announcements about the study; spots on the local network news broadcasts highlighting the services of the center; newspaper articles that discuss the advances in MS and include names of local MS Centers; the Multiple Sclerosis Society's newsletter, web site, and chapter services mailings; and outreach to nurse colleagues who have contact with people with MS in the emergency room, community, and rehabilitation centers (6).

Selecting appropriate patients for a specific clinical trial is a primary nursing focus. In MS trials, it is particularly important to note documented evidence of a diagnosis of MS, exclusionary medications, and the ability to perform outcome measurement tasks, such as a nine-hole peg test. If the trial involves an injectable drug, the patient must be able to learn to self-inject or have a reliable caregiver who is willing to perform the procedure. A family member or significant other should be included during the review of the informed consent form and all education sessions to ensure adherence to the relevant protocol. The use of safe and appropriate assistive devices for mobilizing, along with provisions for adequate transportation, are other nursing considerations when selecting patients for clinical trials.

Nursing assessment of a patient's motivational level and readiness to participate is an important key to selecting appropriate candidates for a study. Questions to ask yourself regarding a patient's motivation include:

+   How realistic are the patient's expectations of what the drug under investigation will and will not do for MS?
+   Does the patient understand that the chance of receiving a placebo exists?
+   Is the patient committed to the frequency of visits, the testing requirements, and the procedures outlined in the protocol?
+   How successful has the patient been in the past? Does he keep scheduled clinical appointments and adhere to therapeutic regimens?
+   Does the patient lack appropriate insurance for available treatment?
+   Is the patient experiencing a decline in functional status despite aggressive therapeutic interventions?

Readiness can be assessed by questioning the patient's availability and by reviewing his vacation plans and work and school schedules. A patient can be highly motivated but simply not ready to enter a trial because of other commitments.

Patient Retention

It can be difficult to keep patients motivated and interested in trials, especially when the study lasts several years. Some of the strategies that are useful in everyday practice and that help to build a reputable MS Center are also important in clinical trial work.

A hospitable environment makes all the difference when caring for people with MS. Patients and families look forward to seeing a friendly face and are comforted by the nurse's presence. A warm hello, a gentle touch, and a comforting conversation help to bring patients back to the study site. Sweets on the desk, flowers in the waiting room, and photographs of family, staff, and vacation spots are just a few props that make the study site more welcoming.

It is important to remind patients participating in a trial that healthcare provisions are available. Rehabilitation, home care, counseling, and medical consultations are just a few of the ongoing services available on-site or by referral to appropriate community resources.

Congratulate patients on their contribution to a greater good. It is important to periodically thank volunteers for their effort and willingness to advance science and to help others with MS. This empowers patients to look at the study as an opportunity that may change their future, as well as the future of all people diagnosed with MS.

Sending holiday, birthday, wedding, anniversary, and sympathy cards is a thoughtful way to reach out to participants. Sponsors often will underwrite this effort if they are approached early in the study.

Frequent telephone contact helps patients maintain a sense of connectedness and provides an opportunity for the nurse coordinator to review protocol issues and screen for adverse events. A call to remind patients of follow-up visits helps to reduce the incidence of "no-shows" and protocol violations.

Patients and family members develop a trusting relationship with the nurse coordinator. Changing a coordinator mid-trial may affect a patient's performance and disrupt the integrity of a study.

Sponsors often offer an open-label extension to the protocol. This allows participants who have successfully completed the double-blind phase to receive drugs free of charge. This motivates patients to continue in a study and is a helpful retention tactic.

Study participants make many mistakes: They forget to bring in unused drug, they forget to call you if there is an adverse event, they take the study drug incorrectly, and they sometimes want to drop out of the trial. A sense of humor and a nonjudgmental approach by the nurse help to minimize a patient's guilt and sense of failure. Humor and unconditional understanding are key elements in retaining patients and ensuring quality in a clinical trial.

Finally, a nurse who is flexible and accommodating will be successful in retaining patients in a clinical trial. Making schedules with patients and families that take into account work, traffic, and parking restraints helps to ease anxiety and reduce stress. A home visit when an unusual situation prevents a visit to the study site demonstrates the importance of the data collected, the value of each participant, and the commitment of the team to quality research.

Hope versus False Hope

Participants have high hopes when they enter a study. Each person expects that the drug will be beneficial and that he will improve. Setting realistic and tangible expectations helps to dilute a sense of false hope. For example, not all participants in a double-blind study receive the study drug, and the drug under study may not be beneficial. Patients must be helped to understand that trial participation is a chance to make a difference in their lives, and that there are options. Patients have the right to withdraw at any point in a study without fearing that their care will be compromised. Recent study designs have included escape clauses that provide parameters for clinicians to prescribe available treatments if the disease is worsening during a trial.

Nurses can share their sense of personal hope with patients and families. Remember that people borrow from a nurse's wellspring of hope (5). Participants sometimes become disheartened and dispirited during a clinical trial because their condition worsens or they believe that they are not receiving the active drug. The nurse's commitment, support, and unending encouragement help restore a sense of hope that sustains a patient throughout a trial. A nurse's hopefulness often is the energy that propels a trial to completion.

There are times when an MS trial goes poorly and patients seem to be worsening. A nurse's sense of hope can be diminished, and guilt feelings may prevail. Reaching out for support from nurse colleagues and other members of the research team can renew the nurse's sense of well-being and hope.

Adherence, Fatigue, Cognition, and Quality of Life Issues

Adherence to the protocol is a tedious task for patients and requires the persistent support of nurse coordinators. Educating patients at the start of the study and reinforcing information throughout is an important intervention to promote adherence to the protocol. A spirit that instills a sense of shared experience and views the patient, family, and research team as part of a collaborative effort helps to ensure adherence (see Chapter 7).

Fatigue is a patient care issue specific to MS and is an important factor in research trials. A patient's energy level and endurance should be considered when planning the order of testing during a visit (e.g., should the patient do the 500–meter walk first or sit for cognitive testing first?). Individual preferences and abilities should be evaluated and addressed during the visit. Nurses should plan rest periods and have cold water and ice packs available to help patients cope with fatigue.

Cognitive impairment in MS can manifest as memory problems, attention deficits, inability to concentrate, or poor judgment (see Chapter 11). Clean, concise, and simply written instructions given in the presence of a caregiver are a key element in protecting patients' rights and maintaining the integrity of the study protocol.

Quality of life during study participation takes on a new meaning. The anticipation of a positive outcome, the well-known placebo effect (7), and the contribution to a greater good give study participants a chance to enhance their quality of life and improve the quality of life for all people with MS.

Food and Drug Administration Audits

Clinical trials are subject to audits by the FDA in order to validate therapeutic claims made by the study's findings (8). The FDA approves a new drug or a new device based on data that are statistically significant and have been obtained in accordance with all rules and regulations.

Good nursing practice is the key to surviving an FDA audit. Accurate, complete, and up-to-date documentation of the events related to the patient's progress throughout the study helps validate any information that has been recorded and sent to the sponsor. An organized and current regulatory file that includes all the items noted in Table 9-1 will withstand an FDA inspection. Honesty and simplicity are the elements required when answering the inspector's questions or concerns. The purpose of an FDA audit is not to find fault or to blame; everyone makes mistakes, and clinical trial work is no exception. Proper documentation and explanation of protocol violations or other deviations protect the integrity of the study. Remember that the FDA is responsible for ensuring that any drug or device that is approved is safe for use in a larger population. The conduct of the study in accordance with FDA regulations and standards ensures that the product was investigated under scrupulous circumstances.

Lisook (8) identified the most common deficiencies found in a sample of over 2,000 FDA audits:

+ Problems with consent forms
+ Protocol nonadherence
+ Inadequate drug accountability
+ Inadequate and inaccurate records
+ IRB problems:
  — No approval
  — Not informed of protocol changes
+ Nonlisting of subinvestigators and/or inappropriate delegation of authority
+ Nonavailability of records
+ Failure to obtain consent

Summary: Recommendations for Research Nurse Coordinators

+ Remember: a study has a beginning, middle, and end; there will be closure.
+ Study work will certainly satisfy a compulsive edge if you have one.
+ Keep in touch with other nurse coordinators for support and information: Sharing experiences is important for everyone's success.
+ Take care of yourself; study work is tiring and stressful. Incorporate ways to relax and re-energize.
+ Enjoy the investigator's meeting—the sponsor is eager to impress investigators and often puts together an elaborate event in a nice location.
+ Think of research questions you may want to incorporate into the study: Sponsors often are willing to listen to a proposal and offer support.

Acknowledgment

The author acknowledges the support and guidance of her first CRA, Jean Peacock.

REFERENCES

1.   Whalen M, Fedor C. Clinical research coordinators: careers and trends. *The Monitor*. 2005; 19(4):23–25.
2.   McGuire Dunn C, Chadwick G. *Protecting Study Volunteers in Research: A Manual for Investigative Sites*. Boston, MA: CenterWatch, Inc., 1999.

3. Iber F, Riley W, Murray P. *Conducting Clinical Trials*. New York: Plenum Publishing, 1987.

4. Rusinek E. Safeguarding human subjects of medical research: control by committee. *Res Nurse*. 1996;2(3):1–9.

5. Steger K. Recruitment of subjects in clinical trials. *Res Nurse*. 1997;3(6):1–12.

6. Costello K, Morgante L, Miller C. The role of the nurse in clinical trials. Workshop presentation, The Consortium of MS Centers Annual Meeting, Cleveland, Ohio, October 3, 1998.

7. Talbot M. The placebo prescription. *New York Times Magazine*. January 9, 2000; 34–29,44,58–60.

8. Lisook A. FDA audits of clinical studies: policy and procedures. *J Clin Pharmacol*. 1990; 30:296–302.

9. Morgante L. Integrating the concept of hope into clinical practice. In: Halper J, Holland N, eds. *Comprehensive Nursing Care in Multiple Sclerosis*, 2nd ed. New York: Demos, 2002.

CHAPTER 10

Case Management

June Halper

Multiple sclerosis (MS) is a chronic, lifelong illness of young adults that requires a wide and variable array of programs and services throughout a lifetime. The continued growth of managed care in the United States and the movement toward integrated delivery networks impel the MS clinical nurse to take on the new and challenging role of case manager. The focus of case management has been defined as the delivery of healthcare that values prevention, early intervention, continuity of care, commitment to quality care, and patient satisfaction (1).

In reality, case management has emerged as a core strategy for cost containment by the managed care industry, emphasizing coordination of services and avoidance of fragmentation and duplication of services (2). In this author's opinion, this approach often fails to adequately consider the needs of people with MS and the reality of the variable challenges of their condition. In the ideal situation, the successful case manager assists patients and their families to access and use relevant resources at the appropriate times and locations (3), despite constraints of the system. Thus, the nurse case manager in MS may also be required to assume an advocacy role to ensure patients' full access to services that are medically, socially, and economically necessary.

The President's Commission on Mental Retardation adopted the concept of case management over 30 years ago (3). This concept has grown to include acute and chronic illnesses, injury and trauma, and worker's compensation cases. Case managers are employed by insurance companies, organizations that subcontract to the insurance industry, and other organizations whose goal is managing spiraling costs in healthcare. They may or may not have a nursing background or, in the case of MS, be familiar with chronic illness and/or physical disability.

Case Management Models

The Case Management Society of America has defined case management as a "collaborative process which assesses, plans, and implements, coordinates, monitors, and evaluates options and services to meet an individual's health needs" (4). Most models and programs focus on a specific patient population through an entire episode of illness (5). These models may be classified as either patient-focused or system-focused (3). The former model emphasizes the relationship of the patient and the case manager; the latter focuses on the service environment, organizational structure, and resource base (6). Patient-focused models are driven by the need for continuity of care, accessibility of healthcare providers, and interdependence between the patient and family and the case manager. On the other hand, system-focused models have increasingly been used for a variety of reasons, particularly for those patients who have not responded well to treatment (7). This model employs critical pathways and disease management teams to meet the episodic needs of a specific group of patients, their disease, and their treatment regimen. Unlike patient-focused models, this model focuses on organizational needs and reimbursement rates as its underlying structure and with its raison d'être being cost containment.

The social service model of care delivery is driven by a philosophy of wellness and health, and was first articulated in the early 1980s for mental health services. Although its original focus was to provide services to the mentally ill to enable them to live independently in the community, its precepts can be readily transferable to the chronically ill or physically disabled (7). The goal of this model was to reduce the risk of long-term institutionalization or acute hospital care. This model was found to be extremely effective in assisting patients to obtain additional benefits, such as Social Security and Medicaid, providing social support through case manager–patient interactions, strengthening existing friend and family ties, and sustaining a supportive social environment (3). It also was found to be effective in maintaining patients' physical health (8), a model particularly relevant to MS care.

Outcomes of Case Management

The literature supports the view that case management can improve healthoutcomes and facilitate cost containment. Gonzalez-Calvo and coworkers (2) concluded that there was significant correlation between case management interventions and problems solved. In their study, planned interventions resulted in good birth outcomes in a high-risk group. Additional studies evaluating the effect of nursing case management on the chronically ill demonstrated a significant decrease in inpatient and emergency visits and reduced lengths of stay in acute-care facilities (9).

Advanced Practice Nursing Case Management Models

During the past decade, nursing has responded to this new challenge by developing nursing practice models based on the case management concept. The value of this trend is the emphasis on nursing leadership and clinical expertise, as demonstrated by several theoretical models that are employed in daily practice (3). The Primm model of differentiated case management, the Star case management model, and the professional nursing case management model are current paradigms of effective case management.

Primm's model of differentiated case management (DCM) is based on the relationship between the patient and the case manager, in which the nurse is accountable for patient care. This model is patient-focused, and all patients are case-managed (3). Nurses are either case managers or care associates based on levels of educational preparation. Case managers develop care plans and are accountable for all aspects of care during hospitalization, whereas care associates implement the plan of care in collaboration with their management colleague. Roles within this model encompass that of consultant, researcher, care provider, and evaluator. Using this model, lengths of stay have been shown to decrease an average of 1.4 days over a 2-year period (10).

The Star model expands on the traditional model incorporating the triad of family, physician, and third-party payers. The advanced practice nurse case manager in this model integrates the needs of the patient, the family's resources, the ability to use community resources, the treatment required, and available coverage into a realistic plan of care (11). This practice model can be used in a home care setting, in an outpatient program, or by an insurance company (11). Although there have been no outcome studies to support sustained long-term benefits, it can be assumed that there will be a natural "fit" in a comprehensive care approach to MS.

St. Mary's Hospital in Tucson, Arizona, approached the challenges of the current healthcare systems with the professional nursing case management model. This model is based on the development of a relationship between the patient, family, and other healthcare participants (11,12). The distinctive roles in this approach involve the integration of nursing services across the care continuum, with a community component that facilitates the nurse to move from the acute care setting into home care and the community. The nurse case manager is responsible for the quality of care, its cost-effectiveness, and reasonable access to healthcare. The process features specific interventions focused on a plan of care that values the patient's illness experiences and include "telling the story," advancing the plan, maintaining values and beliefs, and assisting with options and decisions (12). Implementation of this model has resulted in substantial cost savings in one facility (13). Future studies are required to replicate and support this result in MS and in other chronic illnesses.

Roles and Responsibilities of Case Managers

Although there has been a dearth of research and some debate in this area, a review of the literature reveals the following common functions and responsibilitiesrequired of successful case managers (14):

- Patient identification and outreach
- Individual assessment and evaluation
- Service planning and resource identification
- Linking patients to needed services
- Service implementation and coordination
- Monitoring service delivery
- Advocacy (15)

The successful case manager is required to possess a variety of skills, which should include comprehensive assessment, creative planning, innovative interventions, and negotiation. Personal attributes should include good communication skills, flexibility, sound clinical judgment, and awareness of ethical issues (16). Effective case managers in MS are identified as nurses who are experts in the conduct of comprehensive case management functions that involve direct care, expert guidance and coaching, consultation, interpretation and use of research, collaboration, change agency, and ethical decision making (14). The advanced practice nurse's unique educational preparation provides the underpinnings for the development of a structure that ensures a continuum of care and empowers the patient to assume an active role in his healthcare (3).

Comprehensive Case Management in Multiple Sclerosis

Successful case management in MS must include core nursing components such as assessment, planning, implementation, and evaluation, but also should consider variables such as cultural sensitivity, consumer involvement, payer constraints, and the multidisciplinary approach. The development of this model is a response to the challenges and shortcomings of previously cited models (3) as well as the recognition of the complex and dynamic nature of the disease. The focus on patient empowerment and quality of care is a fundamental principle of this model. It is evident that there is a shift from task orientation to an emphasis on physical and psychological outcomes. These outcomes are the result of a multidisciplinary team approach and statistical analysis to monitor and manage patients and their needs (3). Outcomes include the establishment and attainment of short- and long-term goals appropriate to each patient; they reflect the result of sensitive interactions with the healthcare system.

Heath and coworkers (17) noted the following factors, which should guide patient outcomes: (a) changes in health status; (b) changes in knowledge, which may influence future health; (c) changes in behavior, which may influence future health; and (d) patient and family satisfaction (3). Outcomes offer very useful information about the effectiveness and sustained benefit of healthcare interventions.

Another aspect of comprehensive case management is based on the interdisciplinary approach, a team model that has been found to be appropriate in caring for patients with MS. Team building implies the collaborative efforts of professionals seeking to combine the perspectives of all members into one service and one unified plan. This entails the following:

- Incorporating nursing, social services, and various other health professionals into the service delivery system
- Strengthening and facilitating existing social supports
- Empowering the patient toward self-care
- Promoting communication that supports family-centered care and collaborative, interdependent relationships
- Ensuring the process of the patient's culture, socioeconomic circumstances, and lifestyle (3)

Patient empowerment requires education, networking, skill development, early disease interventions, and a focus on wellness rather than illness. This empowerment model helps patients to recognize their strengths and internal resources, and it can be defined as the "cornerstone of case management" (3).

Incorporating the Model into Multiple Sclerosis Nursing Practice

The comprehensive case management model can be incorporated into MS care in the outpatient, acute care, rehabilitation, and long-term care settings. The nurse case manager enters the system at the time of diagnosis, providing education about the disease, exploring treatment options, and assisting the patient and family to gain access to the medical system. Entry into and maintaining contact with community systems is an important facet of MS case management, and it has been stated that the success of a case manager depends not on the specific model but on the right person with the right training (18).

The advanced practice nurse in MS brings a scope of expertise that encompasses patient and systems advocacy, crisis intervention, home visits, outreach and assessment, practical counseling, and innovative collaboration with both formal and informal systems (3). Adeptness between case management roles requires the synthesis of practical planning, clinical judgment combined with financial responsibility, utilization review, and sustaining care. The roles of a case manager require a knowledgeable nurse who is able to perform in autonomous practice and accept the broad responsibilities involved in the complex environment of MS care. Advanced practice nurses have been found to facilitate both quality care and cost-effectiveness in other chronic illnesses (19) and have emerged as mainstays in comprehensive MS care.

The International Organization of MS Nurses has identified a case management model as a stage-by-stage process (20). Contributors defined the needs of people with MS as differing depending on their specific diagnosis and the course of their illness, with some overlap in newly diagnosed people, those with relapsing-remitting disease, worsening forms of the illness, and those who have advanced MS. During the period of the new diagnosis, the emphasis should be on providing education and information relevant to each person, with the goal to promote the transition to a chronic illness. For those with relapsing-remitting MS (RRMS), based on evidence, interventions included the use of disease modification, relapse management, and symptomatic care. Worsening MS calls for more care planning, more frequent contacts, and concrete services along with environmental changes to adapt to altered functioning. In advanced MS, the need for supportive care included prevention of complications, team management with a medical team and, at times, palliative care (20).

Summary

Case management continues to evolve as a model of care delivery with significant relevance to chronic illness and disability, specifically MS. The process of developing and implementing a comprehensive plan represents an acceptable, dynamic, and pragmatic approach to the delivery of services within the complex and variable circumstances proscribed by this disease. The advanced practice nurse in MS care can sustain and expand this role within complex healthcare delivery systems throughout the world.

REFERENCES

1. Kaluzny AD, Shortell SM. Creating and managing the future. In: Shortell SM, Kaluzny AD, eds. *Essentials of Healthcare Management*. Albany: Delmar Publishers, 1997.

2. Gonzalez-Calvo J, Remington NS, Woodman C, et al. Nursing case management and its role in perinatal risk reduction: Development, implementation, and evaluation of a culturally competent model for African American women. *Public Health Nursing*. 1997;14(4):196–206.

3. Taylor P. Comprehensive nursing case management: An advanced practice model. *Nursing Case Manag*. 1999;4(1):2–10.

4. Tinidad EA. Case management: A model of CNS practice. *Clin Nurse Specialist*. 1993;7(4):221–223.

5. Bower K. *Case Management by Nurses*. Washington, DC: American Nurses Association, 1992.

6. Stahl DA. Case management in subacute care. *Nurs Manag*. 1996;27(8):20–22.

7. Brindis CD, Theidon KS. The role of case management in substance abuse treatment services for women and their children. *J Psychoactive Drugs*. 1997;20(1):79–88.

8. Oriol MD. One agency's formula. *Home Healthcare Nurse*. 1997;20(1):505–508.

9. Huggins D, Lehman K. Reducing costs through case management. *Nurs Manag*. 1997;28(12):34–37.

10. Brubakken KM, Janssen WR, Ruppel DL. CNS roles in implementation of a differentiation case management model. *Clin Nurse Specialist*. 1994;8(2):69–73.

11. Glettler E, Leen MG. The advanced practice nurse as case manager. *J Case Manag*. 1996;5(3):121–126.

12. Forbes MA. The practice of professional nurse case management. *Nurs Case Manag*. 1999;4(1):28–37.

13. Sohl-Kreiger R, Lagaard MW, Scherrer J. Nursing case management: Relationships as a strategy to improve care. *Clin Nurse Specialist*. 1996;10(2):107–113.

14. Mahn VA, Spross JA. Nurse case management as an advanced practice role. In: Hamric AB, Spross JA, Hanson CM, eds. *Advanced Nursing Practice: An Integrated Approach*. Philadelphia: WB Saunders, 1996.

15. Allred CA, Arford PH, Michel Y, et al. The relationship between structure and environment. *Nurs Economics*. 1995;13(1):32–51.

16. Schraeder C, Britt T. The Carle clinic. *Nurs Manag*. 1997;28(3):32–34.

17. Heath II, McCormack B, Phair L, Ford P. Developing outcome indicators in continuing care: Part I. *Nurs Stand*. 1996;10(46):41–45.

18. Brown L, Deckers C, Magallanes A, et al. Clinical case management: What works, what doesn't. *Nurs Manag*. 1996;27(11):28–30.

19. Macias C, Farley OW, Jackson R, Kinney R. Case management in the context of capitation financing: An evaluation of the strengths model. *Admin Policy Mental Health*. 1997;24(6):535–543.

20. Costello K, Halper J, Morgante L, Namey M, contributors. *Case Management in Multiple Sclerosis*. New Jersey: International Organization of MS Nurses, 2005.

CHAPTER 11

Recognizing and Treating Cognitive Impairment

Colleen Murphy Miller

Cognitive impairment may be one of the most feared symptoms of
multiple sclerosis (MS) because it can result in the inability to make
reasonable decisions, manage simple tasks, and remember information that is vital
to all aspects of a person's life. It can change the personality and, in the extreme,
lead to total functional dependence. Unfortunately, there is no proven medical
treatment to reverse the cognitive impairment in MS (1), although there is some
indication that medicines used to treat dementia may also have a desirable clinical
effect in MS patients (2). Recognition of the symptom of "cognitive fatigue"
lends further hope toward a treatment that may improve this type of impairment
(3–5). An emerging body of evidence suggests that the medicines that affect
relapses, inflammation, and the underlying mechanisms of disease may be related
to improvement in neuropsychological function (6–9). Pediatric MS, with its
implications of cognitive impairment among developing children, presents newly
appreciated challenges to nurses and the care team (10).

Nurses are frequently the first and most consistent contact that the person
with MS and her family members have with the healthcare system. Although
they are not the definitive experts regarding cognitive issues, nurses are in a

position to evaluate, communicate with, teach, counsel, and treat patients with these impairments. Multiple sclerosis nurse experts develop insight and special skills in their repeated interactions with cognitively impaired patients. This chapter discusses the nurse's role in caring for the cognitively impaired MS patient and defining effective nursing strategies.

Cognitive impairment in MS relates to the inability to think, remember, and reason logically (11). The specific functions affected by demyelination and axonal loss include memory, attention, information processing speed, comprehension, word finding, visual perception, visual construction, abstract reasoning, and executive functions (12,13). Although historically not appreciated in the literature, prevalence estimates indicate that approximately 40% to 70% of those diagnosed with MS will experience cognitive symptoms. These symptoms most often result in mild to moderate impairment, and can vary from person to person as well as within an individual throughout the course of the illness. They can occur independently of physical deficits and may appear early in the disease process (14). As many as 20% of people with MS suffer from cognitive deficits severe enough to interfere with social relationships and the ability to work (15,16).

The nurse plays a crucial role in the care of the person with MS who displays signs of cognitive impairment. The first nursing intervention must be to establish a relationship based on trust with the patient and her support network. Patients may not be aware that they are experiencing cognitive difficulties, and families may be unaware that certain intolerable behaviors of the person with MS may be related to cognitive dysfunction (e.g., the person with MS who appears giddy and unconcerned about behaviors that have put her and others at risk of physical harm, such as running a red traffic light and causing a car accident). Families may regard the behavior as unacceptable and blame the person for making a wrong decision. A decision such as running a red light demonstrates impaired judgment and may occur because the person with cognitive dysfunction is not able to quickly solve the problem of what to do when the traffic light turns yellow. In the current example, the nurse must guide the patient and family to the realization that a cognitive dysfunction may actually exist, and she must provide information regarding safety issues (17).

Once the nurse has established a relationship, he continues to observe and assess the patient and her interactions. The nursing focus then turns to facilitating communication. When cognitive dysfunction is subtle, the behaviors of the person who is cognitively impaired may produce considerable strain on the social network. The nurse may be in an optimal position to facilitate communication and acceptance. The Multiple Sclerosis Neuropsychological Screening Questionnaire (MSNQ) is a simple tool that can be used in the clinical setting as a preliminary screen for cognitive impairment (18). This 15–item Likert-type scaled questionnaire should be administered to both the patient and a care partner when possible. On occasion, the scores derived from the care partner raise more concern about the presence of cognitive challenges, whereas the responses from the patient may fall in the normal range. Depressed patients tend to over-score their cognitive difficulties, as may those who experience significant fatigue (19). This tool, although very helpful for simple screening, does not replace the evaluation by a neuropsychologist expert in the field of MS care. Formal testing by a neuropsychologist may be necessary to diagnose the impairment, identify comorbidities, and recommend treatment strategies. Documenting the cognitive disability may also be necessary for the purpose of obtaining vocational rehabilitation or applying for disability benefits.

Imaging studies may raise suspicion or be helpful in verifying those structural and functional changes that are correlated with cognitive dysfunction. Conventional magnetic resonance imaging (MRI) measures such as T2 lesion load, gadolinium enhancement, T1 lesion volume, gray matter atrophy, third ventricular width, and whole-brain atrophy have been associated with cognitive decline (20). Evolving imaging techniques such as magnetization transfer imaging (MTR) demonstrate the severity of tissue damage even in the normal-appearing brain (21). Functional MRI (22,23) and positron emission tomography (PET) have been used to document brain activity on a cellular level (24). MRI lesion burden in specific areas of the brain, such as the frontal lobes, has also been correlated directly with cognitive dysfunction (25,26). Cortical atrophy, MR spectroscopy, and diffusion-weighted imaging are currently under investigation as possible measurements of MS disease burden.

Once a cognitive deficit is identified, the nurse can assess the patient's daily routine and design strategies to help the patient and family cope with the disability. For those patients with mild impairment, simple strategies such as reminder notebooks and detailed lists of tasks to be performed may address the problem sufficiently. Those with more advanced decline may require referral for formal cognitive training by a neuropsychologist or a speech and language pathologist. A common problem for the cognitively impaired person with MS is the lack of insight into her limited ability to solve problems and avoid common dangers. Driving safety is a concern that must be considered, requiring formal testing by predriving and driving professionals. Other safety concerns include cooking and impulsive risk-taking behaviors. The cognitively impaired parent of small children presents an array of safety concerns for the children as well as the patient. Cognitively impaired patients with MS are especially vulnerable to abuse because they may not have the capacity to recognize inappropriate advances or to set limits on the behaviors of others. The nurse is obligated to be watchful of conditions that may indicate a potential for abuse and to report to the healthcare team or the authorities any suspicious behaviors or physical signs. The person who is cognitively impaired as a result of MS may have difficulty learning new information and skills. She may also be less flexible because of the challenge of adapting to changed circumstances in social and work roles. Old behaviors that are firmly ingrained can present barriers to modifying lifestyle, managing symptoms, integrating new treatment regimens, and so forth.

The Impact of Cognitive Impairment

Although cognitive impairment may be devastating in regards to employment and social function (16,27), it may not necessarily impact perceived quality of life (28). Patients with cognitive impairment present a major challenge to the clinical team, one that requires patience and persistence. Nurses experienced in the care of cognitively impaired MS patients are quick to recall the difficulties that these patients have in adhering to treatment plans. The cognitively impaired person may need additional reminders to perform procedures such as taking medications. As a result of cognitive impairment, she may be unable to follow through with treatment regimens. Once the problem becomes evident, the nurse must identify a support person to monitor and assist the patient to promote adherence to treatment. A cooperative and available family member should be considered first. Other supports may include a neighbor, friend, or visiting nurse. Unfortunately, evidence suggests that patients with cognitive dysfunction have more unstable family relationships and fewer supportive resources as a result of altered communication patterns and social isolation. They also have less than optimal interactions with clinic personnel and more difficulty adhering to treatment regimens than do MS patients with motor deficits (29). Recent evidence suggests that day treatment programs providing a supportive social environment may improve adherence and enhance the patient's community resources.

Routine daily activities can present a major dilemma for the cognitively impaired MS patient. Difficulties with memory and attention interfere with learning a new task, such as following a recipe. Such impairments may make following the plot of a movie or reading a book very difficult. Memory deficits may make it impossible to remember appointments, and may cause the patient to lose objects such as house keys and wallets. Additionally, memory deficits may make cognitive interventions ineffective if the patient cannot understand the actual prompt to refer to her memory notebook or even how to use the notebook once it is open.

Reduced concentration and attention leads to difficulties learning new tasks or performing multiple activities at one time, as is often required in daily life. Impaired ability to rapidly process new information leads to difficulties in a busy work or home environment. MS patients with cognitive deficits may have subtle problems synthesizing and prioritizing new information such as the pediatrician's directions to give a child antibiotics on an empty stomach. Multiple reinforcements of important information, such as written instructions from the practitioner and pharmacist, are helpful. Although not as obvious as memory deficits, impaired concentration and attention may appear to be a lapse in judgment (30) and may be misinterpreted as deliberate on the part of the patient, thus accentuating social strain.

Word retrieval may be a more obvious problem because it presents with the "tip-of-the-tongue" phenomenon. Those affected have difficulty finding the words they need to communicate their thoughts. They know what it is they want to say, but they cannot find the specific words they want to use. Although frustrating and embarrassing, the "tip-of-the-tongue" phenomenon can be dealt with by substituting other words or describing an object whose name has escaped.

Visual-spatial organization may present as difficulty reading maps or following constructural directions, such as those required to assemble items that come boxed from the store (30). Patients may also have problems putting away items or organizing storage areas.

Executive functioning is often impaired in people with MS (31), which may be demonstrated by the inability of the patient to regulate her behavior or adapt to new situations and solve problems. A person whose executive functioning is impaired may exhibit inappropriate social conduct, such as acting disinhibited and casual. Adjustment to unfamiliar environments or people may be overwhelming.

These cognitive dysfunctions may severely disrupt the MS patient's life. They also may upset family life and relationships, requiring role changes and many adjustments.

Evaluation of Cognitive Impairment

As the member of the healthcare team with the most frequent patient interaction, the nurse is often the first to recognize a change in cognitive functioning. A patient's family may report changes and provide cues to alert the nurse to impending problems. Cognitive problems are not always obvious to the examiner, particularly if the examination is limited in time or in the opportunity for patient interaction. The Mini-Mental State Examination, although used most often in neurologic settings, is insensitive to the subtle changes that may impair daily function in MS. As a result, cognitive dysfunction may go unrecognized by the treating provider (32).

Although a neuropsychological examination is the most definitive means to diagnose cognitive impairment, it is costly and time-consuming. It should be considered when the dysfunction affects a patient's ability to function effectively at work and home. A neuropsychological examination is also indicated for the patient who seeks vocational counseling to identify employment suitable for her ability. Patients applying for disability benefits because of cognitive limitations are also appropriate candidates. The clinician may identify additional situations that merit a formal evaluation.

Depression may present as cognitive impairment if a patient's symptoms reflect a lack of attention to daily activities and function. A disorganized or disheveled patient is not necessarily cognitively impaired. The distinction between depression or other psychiatric illnesses and cognitive impairment can be very subtle. The neuropsychologist is best equipped to discern these differences. Stress and fatigue also can lead to the impression that a patient is cognitively impaired. Certain drugs such as pain medications, antispasticity agents, antidepressants, corticosteroids, anticholinergics, and tranquilizers produce side effects that further complicate the evaluation.

Patients must be prepared for the neuropsychological examination by a supportive clinician. The nurse should inform patients that the testing may take a long time and that patients frequently think they have done poorly, even if their function is normal. Patients should be well rested and nourished before testing. In addition, the testing must be performed in a comfortably cool environment, so that heat intolerance and weakness do not affect the scores.

Coping with Cognitive Deficits

With the information now available, our primary goal is to prevent cognitive impairment (7). Once established, however, two major approaches are used in cognitive rehabilitation or remediation. One is an attempt to restore lost function through retraining. This is most effective in brain-injured patients and less effective in the cognitive dysfunction associated with MS. A second cognitive rehabilitative approach focuses on compensatory strategies to facilitate activities of daily living. This approach is most effective in the treatment of the MS patient (33). Cognitive rehabilitation for patients with global impairment is generally limited (29), so the focus should be on promoting understanding and designing ways for the patient and her family to cope with deficits.

A variety of strategies are available for coping with cognitive impairment in MS. Organizational strategies such as making lists and using calendars for reminders are helpful for the patient with memory dysfunction. A memory notebook to log daily events and reminders also may be useful. Reducing change by organizing the patient's environment and not altering the basic setup is necessary for the cognitively impaired person, much like a familiar environment is for a blind person.

Open and nonjudgmental discussion about the cognitive dysfunction is important for the patient and family, and a care partner is most helpful in directing the function of a cognitively impaired person. Neuropsychological counseling may improve social behaviors in some patients (34). Because change is part of daily living, it must be introduced slowly, and reminders must be used liberally. The patient should also be kept mentally stimulated to avoid withdrawal from the situation.

When planning a teaching session for a cognitively impaired patient, the nurse must allow adequate time for repetition and reinforcement while avoiding fatigue. Attention should be paid to patient comfort by scheduling teaching early in the day and in an environment that is not too warm, because fatigue and heat intolerance may further impair their cognitive performance. Distractions and overstimulation must be eliminated if the teaching is to be effective. Instructions should be simple, and should include the obvious, such as "turn off the stove." Verbal instructions must be reinforced with written or audiovisual directions. Return demonstrations of skills will help establish whether learned material has been retained.

Summary

Nurses should be aware of the needs of the cognitively impaired patient. Faced with the challenges of such patients, the nurse can exercise his unique abilities and knowledge to provide care to patients and families who need individualized understanding and support. Identifying and addressing factors that influence cognition such as fatigue, concurrent illness, and some medication effects is well within the role of the MS nurse. Among the most helpful strategies the nurse can offer include recognizing the problem, facilitating the diagnosis, developing individualized and dynamic plans of care, and minimizing the impact of cognitive impairment on patients' quality of life.

REFERENCES

1. Bagert B, Camplair P, Bourdette D. Cognitive dysfunction in multiple sclerosis: Natural history, pathophysiology and management. *CNS Drugs.* 2002;16(7):445–455.

2. Krupp LB, Christodoulou C, Melville P, et al. Donepezil improved memory in multiple sclerosis in a randomized clinical trial. *Neurology.* 2004;63:1579–1585.

3. Schwid SR, Tyler CM, Scheid EA, et al. Cognitive fatigue during a test requiring sustained attention: A pilot study. *Multiple Sclerosis.* 2003;9:503–508.

4. Krupp LB, Elkins LE. Fatigue and declines in cognitive functioning in multiple sclerosis. *Neurology.* 2000;55:934–939.

5. Sailer M, Heinze HJ, Schoenfeld MA, et al. Amantadine influences cognitive processing in patients with multiple sclerosis. *Pharmacopsychiatry.* 2000;33:28–37.

6. Fischer JS. Neuropsychological function improves with disease modification. *Presentations in Focus.* 1998;(April 24–May 2):4.

7. Fisher JS, Priore RL, Jacobs LD, et al. Neuropsychological effects of interferon β-1a in relapsing multiple sclerosis. *Ann Neurol.* 2000;48(6):885–892.

8. Zéphir H, Seze J de, Dujardin K, et al. One year cyclophosphamide treatment combined with methylprednisolone improves cognitive dysfunction in progressive forms of multiple sclerosis. *Multiple Sclerosis.* 2005;11:360–363.

9. Pliskin NH, Hamer BS, Goldstein MS, et al. Improved delayed visual reproduction test performance in multiple sclerosis patients receiving interferon β-1b. *Neurology.* 1996;47:1463–1468.

10. Banwell BL, Anderson PE. The cognitive burden of multiple sclerosis in children. *Neurology.* 2005;64:891–894.

11. Schapiro RA. *Symptom Management in Multiple Sclerosis,* 3rd ed. New York: Demos, 1998.

12. Fischer J, LaRocca NG, Sorensen P. Cognition. In: Kalb RC, ed. *Multiple Sclerosis: The Questions You Have—The Answers You Need.* New York: Demos, 1996.

13. Rao SM, Leo GJ, Bernardin L, Unverzagt F. Cognitive dysfunction in multiple sclerosis. I. Frequency, patterns, and prediction. *Neurology.* 1991;41:685–691.

14. Amato MP, Ponziani G, Pracucci G, et al. Cognitive impairment in early-onset multiple sclerosis. *Arch Neurol.* 1995;52:168–172.

15. Beatty WW, Paul RH, Wilbanks SL, et al. Identifying multiple sclerosis patients with mild or global cognitive impairment using screening examination for cognitive impairment (SEFCI). *Neurology.* 1995;45:728–723.

16. Rao SM, Loe GJ, Ellington MS, et al. Cognitive dysfunction in multiple sclerosis. II. Impact on employment and social functioning. *Neurology.* 1991;41:692–696.

17. Schultheis MT, Garay E, Deluca J. The influence of cognitive impairment on driving performance in multiple sclerosis. *Neurology.* 2001;56:1089–1094.

18. Benedict RH, Cox D, Thompson LL, et al. Reliable screening for neuropsychological impairment in multiple sclerosis. *Multiple Sclerosis.* 2004;10(6):675–678.

19. Carone DA, Benedict RH, Munschauer FE 3rd, et al. Interpreting patient/informant discrepancies of reported cognitive symptoms in MS. *J Intern Neuropsychologic Soc.* 2005;11(5):574–583.

20. Benedict RH, Carone DA, Bakshi R. Correlating brain atrophy with cognitive dysfunction, mood disturbances, and personality disorder in multiple sclerosis. *J Neuroimag.* 2004;14:36S–45S.

21. Rovaris M, Filippi. MRI correlates of cognitive dysfunction in multiple sclerosis patients. *J Neurovirol.* 2000;6:S172–S175.

22. Staffen W, Mair A, Zauner H, et al. Cognitive function and fMRI in patients with multiple sclerosis: Evidence for compensatory cortical activation during an attention task. *Brain.* 2002;125:1275–1282.

23. Lazeron RHC, Rombouts SARB, Scheltens P, et al. An fMRI study of planning-related brain activity in patients with moderately advance multiple sclerosis. *Multiple Sclerosis.* 2004;10:549–555.

24. Santa Maria MP, Benedict RH, Bakshi R, et al. Functional imaging during covert auditory attention in multiple sclerosis. *J Neurologic Sci.* 2004;21(18):9–15.

25. Sperling RA, Guttmann CRG, Hohol MJ, et al. Regional magnetic resonance imaging lesion burden and cognitive function in multiple sclerosis. *Arch Neurol.* 2001;58:115–121.

26. Benedict RH, Zivadinov R, Carone DA, et al. Regional lobar atrophy predicts memory impairment in multiple sclerosis. *Am J Neuroradiol.* 2005;26(7):1824–1831.

27. Amato MP, Ponziani G, Siricusa G, Sorbi S. Cognitive dysfunction in early-onset multiple sclerosis. A reappraisal after 10 years. *Arch Neurol.* 2001;58:1602–1606.

28. Benedict RH, Wahlig E, Bakshi R, et al. Predicting quality of life in multiple sclerosis: Accounting for physical disability, fatigue, cognition, mood disorder, personality, and behavior. *J Neurologic Sci.* 2005;231(1–2):29–34.

29. Whitham RH. Cognitive and emotional disorders. In: Herndon RM, Seil FJ, eds. *Multiple Sclerosis: Current Status of Research and Treatment.* New York: Demos; 1994:189–209.

30. LaRocca NG, Kalb RC. Psychosocial issues in multiple sclerosis. In: Halper J, Holland NJ, eds. *Comprehensive Nursing Care in Multiple Sclerosis.* New York: Demos; 1997:83–107.

31. Baso MR, Beason-Hazen S, Lynn J, et al. Screening for cognitive dysfunction in multiple sclerosis. *Arch Neurol.* 1996;53:980–984.

32. Heaton RK, Thompson LL, Nelson LM, et al. Brief and intermediate-length screening of neuropsychological impairment. In: Rao SM, ed. *Neurobehavioral Aspects of Multiple Sclerosis.* New York: Oxford University Press; 1990:149–160.

33. Rodgers D, Khoo K, MacEachen M, et al. Cognitive therapy for multiple sclerosis: a preliminary study. *Alt Ther Health Med.* 1996;2(5):70–74.

34. Benedict RHB, Shapiro A, Priore R, et al. Neuropsychological counseling improves social behavior in cognitively impaired multiple sclerosis patients. *Multiple Sclerosis.* 2000;6:391–396.

CHAPTER 12

Strategies and Challenges in Managing Spasticity

*Jane Johnson, Louise Jarrett,
and Bernadette Porter*

Spasticity is one of the more common symptoms of multiple sclerosis (MS), and in an extensive recent survey 84% of people with MS (*n* = 20,969) reported that spasticity affected their daily life (1). The severity of spasticity ranged from minimal, through mild, moderate, to severe, with the latter categories preventing participation in many daily activities. However, despite this variability in presentation, spasticity can often be managed or minimized and secondary changes avoided. Numerous authors have outlined practical approaches to management, and multidisciplinary clinical guidelines are now available (2,3).

To optimize management, teams must be aware of the underlying physiology of spasticity, its course of development, and its impact on the person (2). How spasticity develops is often individual to each person, can vary over time, and can be unpredictable, but coordinated multidisciplinary teamwork can enable the person with spasticity or their caregivers to develop effective management strategies. Teamwork must be collaborative across secondary, primary, and social care sectors (2), with the person with spasticity central to the planning and decision-making process (4). Poor communication and lack of specialist knowledge can lead to patients experiencing increasing disability as a result of secondary complications such as pressure sores and contractures. Knowledge of spasticity management strategies has become an important part of the nurse specialist role when working with and coordinating services for people with MS.

This chapter explores current knowledge of spasticity, the contribution of multidisciplinary teamwork, and the nurse's role in assessment, measurement, education, and management of spasticity. It describes a range of physical and drug management strategies that may be helpful in managing mild to severe spasticity.

What Is Spasticity?

The term *spasticity* has been widely used by healthcare professionals to describe almost any increase in muscle tone, but the definition of spasticity is much narrower, being described as: "a motor disorder characterized by a velocity-dependent increase in tonic stretch reflexes (muscle tone) with exaggerated tendon jerks, resulting from hyperexcitability of the stretch reflex, as one component of the upper motor neurone syndrome" (5).

To put this in simpler terms, spasticity relates to stiff muscles occurring on activation of the stretch reflex through movement. Recently, the idea of stiffness only occurring in this way has been challenged by a European working group, EU-SPASM, which believes that other components can also contribute to muscle stiffness (6). They suggest that stiffness can occur due to changes in the viscoelastic properties of soft tissues and hyperexcitable activity in other pathways (not just that of the stretch reflex), through cutaneous and proprioceptive influences. The EU-SPASM group offered the following alternative definition:

"Spasticity is disordered sensorimotor control, resulting from an upper motor neurone lesion, presenting as intermittent or sustained involuntary activation of muscles" (6).

This less-specific definition allows other symptoms often associated with spasticity, such as spasms and clonus, to fall under this umbrella term *spasticity*. This is in line with how healthcare professionals have used the term, to describe the combination of symptoms a person may present with related to the symptoms of upper motor neurone syndrome (Table 12-1).

However, it is important that this potential combination of symptoms does not lead to confusion during the assessment and selection of treatments, because different symptoms may require different interventions. For the appropriate management of spasticity, it is vital that each member of the multidisciplinary team, the person with spasticity, and their family and caregivers understand the terminology being used and make sure that all are describing the same symptoms.

TABLE 12-1
Positive and Negative Features of the Upper Motor Neurone Syndrome (8)

Positive	Negative
Spasticity	Weakness
Spasms	Reduced dexterity
Clonus	Reduced postural responses
Associated reactions	
Brisk tendon reflexes	
Positive support reaction	
Extensor plantar reflexes	

Used with permission from 8. Stevenson VL, Marsden JF. What is spasticity? In: Stevenson V, Jarrett L, eds. Spasticity Management: A Practical Multidisciplinary Guide. Oxford: Taylor & Francis, 2006.

Why Does Spasticity Occur?

This section gives a brief overview of the neurophysiology of spasticity and reviews the terminology healthcare professionals and people with spasticity must become familiar with. The reader is referred to other texts for further descriptions of related neurophysiology (7,8).

Spasticity often occurs in the presence of other symptoms, and it is described as one component of upper motor neurone syndrome (Table 12-1) (7,8). The control and regulation of normal skeletal muscle activity involves a complex combination of descending motor commands, reflexes, and sensory feedback from the brain, spinal cord, and peripheral sensation. During normal movement, influences from the cerebral cortex, basal ganglia, thalamus, and cerebellum, traveling via upper motor neurones, adjust, reinforce, and regulate the lower motor neurone. This connects directly via peripheral nerves to the muscle to form smooth, coordinated muscle activity and maintenance of posture. Spasticity and other "positive" features of the upper motor neurone (Table 12-1) occur when there is damage to certain upper motor neurone tracts. This interrupts the regulation of spinal cord and lower motor neurone activity, resulting in enhanced lower motor neurone activity and an increase in muscle activity, in response to peripheral stimuli (e.g., muscle stretch, a urinary tract infection, or a pressure sore). In addition, evidence suggests that certain motor neurons serving skeletal muscle are hyperexcitable in spasticity, resulting in muscular contractions from stimuli that would not normally trigger a response (7,8).

Understanding the Terminology

Spasticity relates to muscle stiffness as a result of neural disruption; however, stiffness can also occur independently of this neural component, through immobility and disuse of muscles. These changes can be termed *biomechanical* or *non-neural components*. Non-neural components can lead to intrinsic changes within the muscle and joints, which can cause reduced range of movement and fixed contractures (9).

When a healthcare professional passively moves the limbs of a person with MS, the resistance she feels to this movement is often referred to as *tone*, This is a combination of stiffness from both the neural and non-neural components, and it can range from low (hypotonia), through normal, to high tone (hypertonia).

Spasms are involuntary sudden movements. They can be flexor, extensor, or adductor in nature. Flexor spasms cause a limb to bend upward toward the body, extensor spasms cause a bending away from the body, and adductor spasms cause limbs to move across the body, often seen as a "scissoring" of the lower limbs. The trunk muscles can also spasm, putting the affected person at risk of falling as they arch off the bed or away from the back of a chair.

Clonus is seen as a repetitive involuntary movement, such as the tapping of a foot, often on the footplates of a wheelchair. The terms *spasm* and *clonus* are often used interchangeably, but a clear distinction between them can lead to more effective management.

Associated Symptoms

The management of spasticity is a challenge, not just because of its variability, but because of the potential coexistence of features such as weakness (Table 12-1). It can be difficult for a person to understand that their muscles can be both weak and stiff at the same time, but it is vital to address this if he is to participate in the evaluation and monitoring of drug treatments or strengthening exercise programs.

Pain is also a common feature of spasticity. This can have different features and requires detailed assessment to identify appropriate treatments. Pain associated with spasticity can be described as deep, tugging, or gnawing, particularly at the joints. It is often made worse during spasms and can be relieved with anti-spasticity drugs such as baclofen, tizanidine, or gabapentin. Pain can also occur through muscle disuse, and it may respond to a stretching and exercise program, plus a review of the person's posture and seating. In practice, pain associated with spasticity is often relieved by a combination of these treatments.

Neuropathic pain is often a feature of MS, so it is important to distinguish this from other pain types because the drug treatment is likely to be different.

For example, in the treatment of neuropathic pain, carbamazepine or gabapentin may be useful.

Having outlined the effects of spasticity, it is important to note that it is not always detrimental. Spasticity may improve vascular flow, assist in maintaining an upright posture (10), or be used by some people as a stabilizer on which to stand or walk. Care must be taken when considering treating spasticity, so that the benefits of an individual's spasticity are fully appreciated (11). Detailed multidisciplinary assessment, in which the person with spasticity is central to the decision-making process, is key to devising an appropriate management plan (3).

Impact of Spasticity on Daily Life

Spasticity can impact on all aspects of a person's daily life (2), varying from day to day and sometimes hour to hour. Spasticity and spasms can affect physical ability and safety when walking, transferring, moving in bed, washing, and dressing. Safety in sitting and lying can also be compromised when spasticity limits how effectively a person can be positioned, while sudden spasms or friction on bedclothes or wheelchair footplates can potentially impact on skin integrity and lead to pressure sores (12–14). A combination of poor mobility, dexterity, and lower limb adductor tone may limit indwelling or intermittent self-catheterization management and can severely impact on an individual's sex life. Sleep may be disturbed, causing increased fatigue and other associated factors. Unconventional postures and spasms draw attention to a person's disability, and can have an emotional impact on mood, self-image, and motivation. Increased dependence on others can significantly alter family dynamics, as well as prospects for work and leisure, with potentially profound effects on the quality of life for all those involved.

Because of its complex nature, yielding some benefits to function as well as problems, the aims of treatment are not necessarily the removal of all spasticity. Goals must be directed toward improving function, reducing pain, and preventing complications, with the ultimate aim of increasing quality of life (15,16).

Managing spasticity can be enormously effortful for an individual, his family and caregivers. Sometimes the effort seems to produce little gain, because often this effort is directed at maintaining current levels of function rather than improving it.

The complex spasticity-related problems experienced by many people with MS often call for an integrated team approach across the spectrum of primary, secondary, and social care (2), although in practice many professionals have tended to work in isolation. Managing spasticity is usually ongoing and will involve close liaison between healthcare professionals working in different settings. This said, the majority of the work will be done by the patient or his family and caregivers, with defined periods of input from different team members (4).

It is paramount that the individual with MS—and in many cases his family—receives education about spasticity and the potential treatments available, so that he can play as active a role as possible in its management.

Comprehensive assessment is the starting point to devising an effective spasticity management plan. The following sections outline assessment and the available options for treatment. Where appropriate, the role of the nurse is highlighted alongside the contributions of other members of the multidisciplinary team.

Assessment

Multidisciplinary assessment is the ideal, a situation in which the patient, his family, and caregivers are included in the team and in which the outcome and plan is communicated to all appropriate members involved in care (3). Team members can learn from each other and extend their repertoire of knowledge during such specialist assessments (3). Assessments must be sensitively led, so that the patient can be an active member, not outnumbered or merely a passive recipient of advice. Conversely, some individuals prefer professionals to drive the decision-making process, and this also needs to be carefully negotiated.

Assessment has three main components: a detailed individual history, physical examination, and the recording of potential outcome measures to assess effectiveness of treatments (3).

The History

The history of a patient's spasticity and its context is necessary to help identify the impact this has on his life and that of his family. It can also help to identify potential goals of treatment. It is important to detail what treatments have been tried in the past, their effects, and reasons for stopping the treatments so that new or revised treatment plans can build on previous experience and methods. For example, it is not uncommon for a patient to claim that oral antispasticity drugs did not work but, on closer examination, it becomes apparent that the drugs did indeed reduce spasticity and spasms, but at the same time exposed underlying weakness that hindered function. Careful titration of the drug at lower doses may mean that medications that had been dismissed could be beneficial. Support is often required for the patient to try the drug again if he has a lasting memory of it as a bad experience. However, because the range of oral drugs available to manage spasticity is limited, judicious use of those available is paramount if the patient's confidence is not to be lost. Such education, monitoring, and support can be a clear role for nurses.

Another important area for nurses during the assessment phase is to help the patient establish priorities and realistic goals when managing his spasticity, within the context of his chosen lifestyle. In addition, it is important to assess the impact that spasticity and its treatment may have on the family unit. This is particularly pertinent when considering invasive methods such as intrathecal treatments, because these may create or reduce the workload for the person and his family. However, less invasive treatments can also create disruption to daily routines, and a patient may need support from his family to complete them successfully.

The optimum timing of treatments and education must be considered for each individual. For example, one woman resisted the idea of coming into hospital for an intrathecal baclofen trial until it emerged that her sons were due to sit exams during the time she would be in the hospital. Rescheduling the admission to fit into her role as a mother enabled her to support her sons but also gave her greater space to focus on herself and work in partnership with the team to establish whether the treatment would improve her life or not.

Physical Examination

This part of the assessment involves observation and a subjective assessment of what the patient's spasticity "feels like." While listening to the history of a patient's spasticity, members of the team will also be noting how the patient's body is moving. Are spasms present? What type are they? Do they compromise safety, skin integrity, or present other issues? Is there clonus? What is his posture like in the chair? In the past, these issues may have been seen as the domain of therapists, either physiotherapists or occupational therapists, but it is now recognized that, although different members of a team may ask the same questions or see the same movements, their perspectives and values will differ. For example, when considering a person carrying out a 10-meter walk, a physiotherapist would assess the quality of the movements and try to establish the relative contributions of neural and biomechanical components, whereas a doctor may consider any further pathology that may be impacting on these movements or whether drug interactions are contributing to the overall presentation. The nurse will consider if any stimuli, perhaps from pressure areas or bladder or bowel problems, are likely to affect spasticity levels and therefore impact on walking. The nurse may also be considering what importance walking has for this individual, both practically and emotionally. Nursing skill in assessing the person's skin integrity, nutritional status, and bladder, bowel and sexual function are valuable during these assessments to predict how changes in the level of spasticity might impact on function. The occupational therapist may consider how the person's movements may be hindered or assisted by the environment he lives or works in. Although roles may overlap, the sharing of this information as a team with the patient and his caregivers can provide a comprehensive assessment and enable the development of a realistic management plan.

The second aspect of the physical assessment is to move the patient's stiff limbs and/or trunk. It is not uncommon for a patient to describe his legs as stiff but, when a healthcare professional passively flexes and extends the legs, they are easy to move with no resistance and therefore no evidence of increased tone. Weak legs can be very heavy for a person to move, and he may describe them as stiff, so it is important to establish if true spasticity exists before instigating antispasticity drug management.

Outcome Measures

Spasticity is notoriously difficult to measure, partly because knowledge of spasticity and its definitions are still evolving. Despite this, a plethora of different measures have been devised in an attempt to objectively measure change. Current measures have been reviewed and fall into three different domains (a) clinical (17), (b) biomechanical (18), and (c) neurophysiologic (19).

These reviews highlight that no one measure adequately measures spasticity. What is useful to the scientific community is not necessarily useful in the clinical setting, and none of the commonly used scales assesses the perspective of the person with spasticity. The second point has recently been addressed in the development of a new scale specific to the MS population (The Multiple Sclerosis Society Spasticity Scale, MSSS-88). This 88-item patient-based, interval-level scale not only looks at spasticity symptoms but also incorporates the person's experience of spasticity and its impact (20). It is likely that a battery of measures is needed to adequately assess spasticity. As well as the person's perspective, this battery might include a subjective assessment of tone (21), a spasm frequency scale (22), and numeric visual or verbal analog scores of pain, stiffness, and discomfort (3).

The process of objective measurement of spasticity may be challenging for some individuals. The aim of measurement is to make a judgment. This can bring a patient's level of disability starkly into focus, not just for the healthcare professional but for the person affected and his family members (4). This can trigger a focus on how his body is changing, threatening how he has envisaged himself within the context of his illness (23,24). Being measured can make people feel as if they are being tested. Healthcare professionals must be aware of these issues and use strategies to minimize these feelings for individuals when carrying out measurements. The nurse's supporting and educating role in this issue is vital.

Basic Principles Underlying Management

Based on sound assessment, a management plan, including physical and drug management components, must be de vised. This should take into account certain basic principles:

TABLE 12-2

Cutaneous and Visceral Stimuli That May Aggravate Spasticity or Spasms

Cutaneous Stimuli	Visceral Stimuli
◆ Altered skin integrity — Red or inflamed skin — Broken skin — Infected skin — Pressure sores — Ingrown toenails ◆ Tight-fitting clothes or urinary leg bag straps ◆ Uncomfortable orthotics or seating systems	◆ Any systemic or localized infection ◆ Bowel dysfunction (e.g., constipation, overflow, or diarrhea) ◆ Bladder dysfunction (e.g., infections, retention, or incomplete emptying) ◆ Deep vein thrombosis ◆ Menstruation

◆ *Exacerbating Factors.* Various visceral and cutaneous stimuli (Table 12-2) are known to exacerbate spasticity. Nurses have key skills in managing such stimuli, and are best placed to educate individuals about these effects. The prevention or management of cutaneous and visceral stimuli is the first line of treatment before considering increasing medication. However, occasionally it may be necessary to increase medication for a defined period until these stimuli resolve. For example, one man noticed that he had an increase in spasms coinciding with the discovery of a kidney stone, and he required an increase in his antispasticity medication until he could be admitted to the hospital for treatment of his kidney stone.

◆ *Movement.* Incorporating movement and stretches into daily activities, whether passive or active, is essential at all stages of spasticity management (2). This, together with effective positioning, exercise, standing, and splinting, can help to maintain range of movement and joint alignment by limiting soft-tissue shortening and preventing contractures (25).

Where possible, active movements and exercise to increase strength and cardiovascular fitness should be planned with the advice of a physiotherapist (25). Studies in people with MS have shown strengthening programs have beneficial effects on fatigue, walking ability, and psychological well-being (26). Likewise, a Cochrane review of all available evidence a dvocated exercise as beneficial for people with MS who are not currently experiencing a relapse (27).

Even if requiring considerable aid from supportive devices, standing is highly recommended as a way of stimulating antigravity activity, reducing flexor tone, and maintaining muscle and joint range (28,29). Weight-bearing through the feet, with good limb and body alignment, often reduces tone throughout the rest of the body. Standing is recommended for up to 30 minutes, ideally once or twice a day, as long as the person can tolerate it (30). The choice of standing aids or frames, and the initial establishment of a therapeutic standing program, is best carried out by a skilled physical therapist but may then be maintained by family members, nurses, and caregivers over the longer term (25).

Where exercise and active movements are limited or not possible, it is recommended that limbs are put through their full range of movement at least once a day (25). This is important but can potentially be damaging if not carried out with care. Putting joints through a full range of movement should, when possible, be a dynamic process with the patient's active involvement, rather than performed passively or by electrical stimulation (30). Great care should be taken if the patient is unable to participate or to signify pain due to sensory problems, because vigorous overstretching can cause trauma and exacerbate stiffness in vulnerable joints. Although these movements can be carried out by a trained caregiver, the technique should initially be taught by a physiotherapist.

The use of orthoses or splints may be a useful adjunct to physical therapy treatment, because they can provide a way of controlling the range of movement around a joint, provide a prolonged stretch, and promote comfort (25). However, these aids can have a number of disadvantages. If poorly fitted, they may serve as a resistance against which spasticity increases. They may cause abrasions and pressure sores that will exacerbate spasticity or significantly alter a person's usual dynamic movement, with obvious detrimental effects. Although orthoses are available through shops or catalogs, they should be fitted and assessed by professionals, and people should be discouraged from purchasing them without advice (15).

Patients with spasticity who find movement difficult may find it easier to move and be supported in water, and may benefit from hydrotherapy or swimming (25).

+ Positioning. Optimizing a person's position throughout a 24–hour period is an important principle in the management of spasticity. The effect of positioning can be enhanced when combined with the movements just described. Incorporated into a management plan, the benefits of proper positioning include lengthening of vulnerable soft tissues, correcting asymmetry (particularly of the spine and pelvis), and supporting the body in a comfortable position to allow relaxation.

Patterns of spasticity can be changed and spasms can reduced by postures that work in opposition to the pattern of spasticity or spasms (e.g., if extensor spasms are problematic, then position the limb in flexion) (25).

Equipment such as a profiling bed, wedges, t-rolls, or simply hoisting someone from their chair to the bed may assist in changing a person's pattern of movement and can contribute to preventing secondary complications (14). Lying supine in extension for extended periods tends to exacerbate spasticity, often leading to difficulty with morning transfers. Placing a rolled towel in the small of the back can increase the base of support provided when lying supine. A large base of support encourages relaxation and a general lowering of postural tone, often with positive effects on lower limb spasms and stiffness. Side-lying or the introduction of some flexion at the hips and knees, supported by pillows, also helps break up extensor tone in the legs.

Appropriate seating, especially for wheelchair users, is recognized as of paramount importance in reducing secondary complications and allowing maximum functional independence (31). As a general principle, the aim is a balanced, symmetric, stable posture with hips, knees, and ankles at 90–degree angles (32). The maintenance of this posture may require a variety of seating adjustments and supports and call on the joint skills of the physical and occupational therapists to tailor a chair to an individual's requirements. In addition, many people with MS who have proximal muscle weakness and poor trunk stability experience increased tone in upper and lower limbs while attempting to maintain their posture in sitting or standing. This can be exacerbated by unsupportive seating and some forms of unstable pressure-relieving devices.

Overall, people with MS who have significant disability can be particularly vulnerable to a vicious cycle involving poor positioning, skin breakdown, and increased spasticity. The combination of reduced mobility and sensory impairment can quickly lead to pressure area damage, which in turn exacerbates spasticity. Increased tone may further limit movement and create problems in trying to achieve and maintain effective pressure-relieving positions. In addition, frequent lower limb spasms can cause friction (e.g., against wheelchair footplates) and result in further skin breakdown.

Management Options

An important part of any MS professional's activity is to provide people with MS and their families with specialized knowledge and skills that will enable and encourage self-management. The complexity of problems experienced by many people with MS often calls for an integrated team approach, which may best be provided by a rehabilitation team.

Multidisciplinary Rehabilitation

Rehabilitation is a goal-directed, problem-solving, often educational process whereby an individual with acquired disability regains or develops new abilities and roles in life, often supported by therapists or other rehabilitation professionals.

As shown earlier, team members can make very different contributions to the overall assessment and ongoing management of spasticity. In practice, some of these roles overlap. Conversely, input and expertise from other professionals across health and social services may also be required—for example, from general practitioners, dieticians, continence advisors, community physiotherapists, and specialist seating services. Nurses working in the MS field are in a good position to help coordinate some of this input by virtue of their holistic approach and educative skills (33).

The advent of new drug treatments has created a whole population of people who are relatively well into contact with nurses working in the MS field, providing ideal opportunities for health education at an earlier stage. In terms of spasticity, knowledgeable nurses are able to advise on the avoidance of exacerbating factors, the benefits of movement and appropriate positioning, suggest appropriate referrals, and develop the idea of an ongoing partnership with professionals that may help maintain "wellness" and a sense of control. The principles of rehabilitation underpin most spasticity management strategies described in this chapter, although periods of more coordinated, intensive multidisciplinary rehabilitation may be needed periodically to review and identify new strategies as circumstances change.

Drug Treatment Options

Oral Medications Used in the Treatment of Mild to Moderate Spasticity

The sites of action and mechanisms of drugs used in the treatment of spasticity are not clearly understood, but it is thought that these agents either alter the function of neurotransmitters or modulators in the central nervous system (CNS) or have an action on peripheral neuromuscular sites (34).

Although a number of drugs have been used to treat spasticity, only four pharmaceutical agents are approved by the U.S. Food and Drug Administration (FDA) for the treatment of spasticity related to CNS damage. These drugs—baclofen, tizanidine, diazepam, and dantrolene sodium—are also the mainstay of treatment in Europe.

Baclofen

Gamma-aminobutyric acid (GABA) and glycine are the main inhibitory neurotransmitters in the CNS (15,34). GABA receptors are located on pre- and postsynaptic membranes and have been divided into two main types, $GABA_A$ and $GABA_B$.

Baclofen [4-amino-3 (4-chlorophenol) butanoic acid] is structurally related to GABA. Oral baclofen crosses the blood–brain barrier and binds pre- and postsynaptically with $GABA_B$ receptors, resulting in inhibition of mono- and polysynaptic spinal reflexes and an associated reduction in spasm, clonus, and pain.

Oral baclofen is the most commonly used antispasticity agent. It should be started at a low dose (possibly only 5 mg/day) and gradually increased as tolerated (by 5 mg/week in sensitive patients) until optimum response is achieved. Slow increase is important because patients sometimes refuse to consider baclofen treatment after experiencing side effects from building up the dose too quickly. If problems arise, the patient is advised to go back to the previous dose before attempting a further gradual increase. Baclofen should not be stopped abruptly because sudden withdrawal may result in rebound spasm, hallucinations, or seizures (a reduction of 10 mg/week is recommended). Side effects associated with oral administration of baclofen include hallucination and confusion in the elderly, increased seizure activity in those with epilepsy, and cardiorespiratory depression and coma when given abruptly in large doses. In practice, these side effects can be avoided by careful assessment and titration. Titration is important to ensure that significant muscle weakness does not occur, because many people rely on the increased tone of spasticity to maintain standing and seating posture. The most commonly reported side effect of baclofen is drowsiness, which usually resolves within a few days. The potential of alcohol or other CNS depressants to exacerbate sedation should be explained to the patient in detail.

Several studies give objective evidence of the effect of baclofen in MS. Shakespeare and colleagues (35), Beard and colleagues (36), and Paisley and coworkers (37) showed a significant change in the Ashworth score (21) of patients treated with baclofen, with reduced spasms and increased range of movement reported, although none of the studies reported any measurable effect on function. Three MS studies compared baclofen to diazepam, with no signi ficant difference in effect; however, generally patients preferred baclofen due to its side-effect profile (38–40).

Tizanidine

Tizanidine (Zanaflex) works as an agonist at central 2-adrenergic receptor sites spinally and supraspinally. It causes preferential inhibition of polysynaptic reflexes, in contrast to baclofen, which appears to preferentially reduce mono-synaptic excitation.

There are suggestions that tizanidine causes less muscle weakness than baclofen (35). Studies have demonstrated a beneficial effect of tizanidine in MS-related spasticity (35–37) and, in comparative trials, it demonstrated a similar degree of efficacy to baclofen (41,42).

Tizanidine therapy may be initiated with a single dose of 2 mg at bedtime, and should be titrated upward very gradually. Dose increases of 2 mg each week may be required until achieving a maintenance dose that meets therapeutic goals with minimal side effects. The maximum recommended dose is 36 mg per day.

Side effects include drowsiness, dry mouth, dose-dependent bradycardia, and hypotension. Adverse effects may be minimized by gradual titration and spreading the dose throughout the day. Changes in liver function can occur, so liver function tests are recommended prior to starting treatment and regularly throughout the first 6 months until treatment is stabilized (43).

Diazepam

Diazepam (Valium) is a benzodiazepine that increases the sensitivity of GABA receptors, resulting in enhanced presynaptic inhibition. Diazepam is useful as a single therapy or in combination with other antispasmodic drugs. It is used extensively with good effect in people with spasticity following spinal cord injury, but generally has not been as helpful in those with spasticity of cerebral origin.

Diazepam should be initiated at a low dose of 2 mg twice daily, increasing by 2-mg increments until therapeutic action without side effects is achieved. The maximum dose can be 30 to 60 mg daily (43). The incidence of sedation is more common with diazepam than with baclofen.

The main side effects associated with diazepam include somnolence, dizziness, and excessive muscle weakness. Paradoxical side effects may include insomnia, anxiety, hostility, hallucinations, and physical addiction. However, the central depression caused by diazepam may be useful in controlling spasms that disturb sleep, and it is often prescribed for use at night.

Clonazepam, a related benzodiazepine, seems to be particularly useful for nocturnal spasms and stiffness, with a less marked side-effect profile than diazepam. It can therefore be prescribed in preference to diazepam at night (3).

Dantrolene Sodium

Dantrolene sodium is unique among the antispasticity drugs because it acts on the muscle fiber rather than on the CNS. A number of complex steps are associated with normal muscle contraction and relaxation, in which the movement of calcium plays an important role.

Dantrolene sodium works by inhibiting the release of intramuscular calcium stores from the sarcoplasmic reticulum, thus interfering with the process of muscle contraction. It may be used in conjunction with centrally acting drugs, but its value may be limited because it can exacerbate some of the side effects of these, such as drowsiness. Dantrolene sodium should be started at a dose of 25 mg daily and increased by 25 mg as tolerated to a maximum of 400 mg daily. Because it is metabolized mainly in the liver, tests of liver function should be checked before starting treatment and monitored closely thereafter. Side effects include nausea, vomiting, and excessive muscle weakness; in general, it is very poorly tolerated. If there is no obvious clinical benefit demonstrated within 6 weeks, the therapy should be stopped because of the risk of irreversible liver damage. Dantrolene sodium is not used frequently for MS in North America because of its side effects and potential for hepatotoxicity.

Gabapentin

Gabapentin is a relatively new drug that can be particularly helpful when stiffness and spasms are associated with pain. It was initially launched as an anticonvulsant during the early 1990s, but its main use over recent years has been to relieve neuropathic pain. It has gained favor as an antispasticity agent, a role in which it appears to be a useful adjunct. Its effectiveness is supported by two small, double-blind, placebo-controlled randomized studies in people with MS (44,45). Like baclofen and benzodiazepines, gabapentin is another GABAergic drug; however, it does not bind with either $GABA_A$ or $GABA_B$ receptors. Its specific mode of action is unknown. Generally, gabapentin is well tolerated. Its main adverse effects are drowsiness, somnolence, and dizziness. The dosage regime does allow for a fairly rapid dose titration; however, if side effects occur, this should be slowed down or the total dose reduced (43). The normal starting dose is 300 mg once a day (100 mg daily in susceptible individuals), increasing to 300 mg twice a day and then 300 mg three times a day. Further increments of 300 mg to 600 mg can then be made every few days up to a total daily dose of 2,400 mg per day (43).

Cannabinoids

The main active ingredient of the cannabis plant (*Cannabis sativa*) is delta-9–tetrahydrocannabinol (THC), which is available as a synthetic pharmaceutical product (Marinol). THC is one of over 60 cannabinoids, and its isolation from other cannabinoids may effect its action. For this reason, some studies have used whole-plant extracts (available in the United Kingdom and Canada as an oromucosal spray, Sativex). The brain and spinal cord have cannabinoid receptors of a type called CB1. CB1 is expressed strongly in the cerebellum, hippocampus, and basal ganglia, which partly explains cannabinoids' predominant effect on short-term memory and coordination (46). However, high concentrations of CB1 are also found in the dorsal primary afferent spinal cord regions, where it may exert its effect on pain and possibly spasticity.

There have been anecdotal but well-publicized reports of cannabinoids reducing pain and spasticity in people with MS, with several self-report studies demonstrating improvement in pain, spasms, sleeping, bladder control, and spasticity (47–53). Evidence from one study (53) showed an objective improvement in spasticity, as measured by the Ashworth scale, for THC-treated individuals.

Side effects can include a mildly euphoric state with some psychomotor slowing and cognitive changes particularly impacting on short-term memory. Anxiety, panic, paranoia, and occasional psychosis can also occur. Other effects include appetite stimulation, hypotension, redness of the eyes, dry mouth, and dizziness (43).

Because cognitive dysfunction and depression are common symptoms of MS (54,55), the reports of these symptoms as side effects of cannabis may potentially limit its therapeutic value, and the use of cannabis remains illegal in many countries. Synthetic cannabinoids or pharmaceutical cannabis plant extract are not currently licensed for the management of spasticity in the United Kingdom, although Sativex is available on a named-patient basis. Two synthetic cannabinoids—nabilone (in Europe) and dronabinol (in the United States and Canada)—are approved for prescription. Nabilone was originally designed to help reduce nausea and increase appetite in people receiving chemotherapy, and it may also be used to help control pain. The recommended dose is 1 to 2 mg daily, up to a maximum of 6 mg per day in divided doses. Dronabinol can be started at 2.5 mg and gradually increased as necessary, although side effects of synthetic cannabinoids are reported in approximately half of patients given standard doses. Oral absorption is a less reliable method of delivering a consistent dose than inhalation, because the drug is rapidly degraded by the liver (43).

In summary, anecdotal and some objective evidence points to the cannabinoids' effect on spasticity but more research is required before it can be established as a routine treatment.

Botulinum Toxin

A growing body of evidence demonstrates the effectiveness of botulinum toxin (BTX) in reducing spasticity in the clinical setting (56). Controlled studies (57–65) and uncontrolled studies (58) have demonstrated the benefits of BTX in reducing impairment and, to a more limited extent, in improving activity.

BTX is a powerful neurotoxin that acts by blocking cholinergic transmission at the neuromuscular junction. When it is injected into spastic muscles, it produces local paralysis of those muscles. Intervention with BTX relies on skilled assessment and identification of the spastic muscles, followed by accurate injection of the toxin. When applied in this manner, it can reduce overactivity in the selected muscle, while maintaining strength in other muscles.

Once injected, BTX takes between 3 and 14 days to produce its full effects of weakening or paralysis of muscles, which then lasts for between 2 to 4 months. However, the combination of BTX with concurrent physical therapy may extend the benefits of BTX alone and may often produce a more significant and long-lasting result. Botulinum toxin is licensed for use in focal upper limb spasticity in both the United Kingdom and the United States. It is also widely used in clinical practice in many other presentations of spasticity in the lower limb and also in the head and neck.

Guidelines for the use of BTX in adult spasticity management have been developed in the United Kingdom by a multidisciplinary working party and published by the Royal College of Physicians (66). The guidelines emphasize the importance of physiotherapy and splinting to maintain and prolong the effects of BTX. They also stress the need for multidisciplinary assessment, with identification of agreed-upon goals for intervention and outcome measurement tools to help review them.

Intervention with BTX should be followed by a formal assessment of outcome. This is most appropriately undertaken by a physiotherapist at 1 to 14 days following injection. Further reviews would ideally be undertaken at 4 to 6 weeks and 3 to 4 months by the multidisciplinary team to evaluate the full impact on daily activities (66). Nurses are likely to be involved in identifying patients who may benefit from BTX intervention and in helping review the effectiveness of such interventions, especially when BTX intervention is considered for improving ease of care and maintaining skin integrity, as in the spastic clenched fist or perineal hygiene related to adductor spasticity (67).

Transcutaneous Electrical Nerve Stimulation

Transcutaneous electrical nerve stimulation (TENS) has been mainly used to treat chronic pain syndromes, but it may have beneficial effects on spasticity for some patients, including those with MS (68). Its mode of action appears to be an increase in the production of endorphins, which, being similar in structure and activity to opiates, can exert both analgesic and muscle relaxant effects. Instructions to patients emphasize the need to persevere for at least 2 weeks, applying electrodes over the affected muscle groups for a minimum of 8 hours each day. Further clinical evaluation of this technique is required to establish whether it has a significant role to play in spasticity management, but its simple, noninvasive approach is attractive to some patients.

Medications Used in the Treatment of Severe Spasticity

In general, working through simple noninvasive management strategies should always be considered before invasive and neurolytic treatments. However, for a small group of patients, spasticity becomes too severe to respond to any of the previously mentioned forms of management. In such cases, intrathecal or surgical options may need to be considered.

Intrathecal Baclofen Treatment

The first continuous intrathecal baclofen (ITB) infusion was reported by Penn and Kroin in 1984 (69), and this mode of delivery has been shown to be effective for people with MS (70). It has developed into a technologically advanced treatment for carefully selected people with severe spasticity.

Although extensively used orally, baclofen does not readily cross the blood–brain barrier. Administration directly into the spinal subarachnoid space permits immediate access to the drug receptor sites concentrated around laminae 2 and 3 of the dorsal horn of the spinal cord (71). Intrathecal use permits effective treatment of spasticity with baclofen doses of less than one-one-hundredth of those required orally. In the cerebrospinal fluid (CSF), baclofen has a half-life of 5 hours and a duration of approximately 10 to 12 hours, with very little drug returning to the systemic circulation (72).

Delivery Systems

Implanted pump delivery systems consist of a reservoir connected via a tunneled catheter to the lumbar subarachnoid space (Figure 12-1). Different types of pump are available; some are battery-powered electronic models that can be programmed by a computer using telemetry, which enables the dose to be varied over a 24–hour period. Other pumps use a gas compression reservoir to provide an inexhaustible energy source, thus delivering a constant dose over the 24–hour period. The flexibility of the dosing programs of electronic pumps can be advantageous, particularly in people with MS, because their spasticity can vary during a 24–hour period (73).

The pump is implanted into a subcutaneous abdominal pocket, and the catheter is run into the intrathecal space with the tip situated at L2–L3 or higher. This allows the drug to be delivered directly toward the GABA receptors of the spinal cord. Figures 12-2 and 12-3 are part of the Medtronic SynchroMed Infusion System. This system is externally programmed using a hand-held computer and telemetry (Figure 12-3). A 24–hour dose can have up to ten steps, each prescribing the dose, rate, and duration, thus allowing the delivery of complex regimens. Current models have a battery that depletes after 5 to 7 years, necessitating an entire pump replacement. An alarm system on the pump will alert the user if the reservoir volume is low, the battery depleted, or the pump malfunctions.

Patient Selection

As with any form of invasive treatment, careful patient selection is essential. Agreeing on a goal of treatment between the patient and the team is an effective way to measure the outcome of ITB treatment (70). Goals can be set to improve transfers, reduce pain and discomfort, improve sitting and lying postures, increase ease of using standing equipment, and to improve ease of lower-body hygiene (70).

If the usual noninvasive management strategies have been tried systematically and are no longer effective or indicated, ITB can be considered an option.

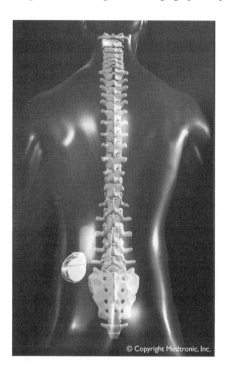

FIGURE 12-1

Site showing placement of an implanted intrathecal baclofen pump. Medtronic SynchroMed Infusion System.

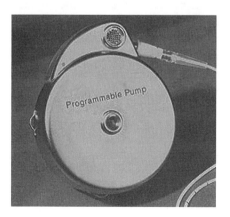

FIGURE 12-2

Medtronic SynchroMed Infusion System pump.

Successful ITB therapy depends on the individual being fully involved in the assessment and selection of ITB as a treatment. Education, including detailed

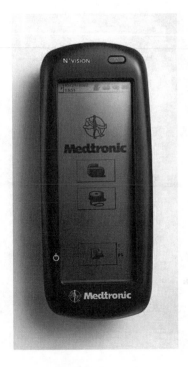

FIGURE 12-3

Medtronic SynchroMed Infusion System hand-held programmer.

explanations of the different stages, the trial, the implant, pump replacement, and ongoing follow-up is integral to the process, and specialist nurses can play a key role. Ideally, verbal explanations should be supplemented with written information or with the use of visual aids such as an imitation pump (73).

The person and/or caregiver should be capable of monitoring and reporting any adverse changes, should understand the risks involved, and must demonstrate commitment to adhere to the therapy.

Following initial selection, a screening phase is necessary to test the degree of response to baclofen delivered intrathecally. Because of the risk of complications, it is recommended that this be carried out in a specialized center where treatment protocols are standardized, full medical support is available, and outcomes can be systematically measured (74). Coordination is the key to an effective ITB management service (75), and a nurse specialist is often in the best position to provide continuity from initial selection to long-term follow-up, supported by appropriate multidisciplinary team members. An outline of the nurse's role in ensuring a safe multidisciplinary ITB service; examples of information leaflets, nursing care plans, and nurse competencies; and associated medical, surgical and physiotherapy protocols and guidelines can be found in Jarrett (73).

The ITB Trial

The trial consists of administering a bolus dose of ITB via lumbar puncture. Some centers suggest performing two trials on separate days to confirm response and gauge the potential for goal achievement (73). The initial dose given is 25 μg, with increments being no more than 25 μg at a time. On rare occasions, if excessive weakness underlying the spasticity is exposed by the 25–μg dose, the second dose is halved to 12.5 μg. This occurs predominantly when the aim is to preserve the quality and ability of the individual to walk or transfer (73). Individuals who do not respond to a 100–μg test dose usually are not considered suitable candidates to proceed, as continuing high-dose delivery in the future is likely to result in unwanted side effects and frequent pump refilling.

This test stage requires vigilance from nursing staff and the availability of respiratory support facilities, because cerebral side effects are most likely to occur following bolus administration (76). Signs of overdose include drowsiness, light-headedness, progressive weakness, decreased respiratory function, and coma. Frequent monitoring of vital signs, oxygen saturation levels, and neurologic status are recommended. Nurses caring for the patient should be aware that drug action tends to peak 2 to 4 hours after injection. The anticholinesterase physostigmine has been used to reverse drowsiness and respiratory depression in cases of mild ITB overdose, but this is short-acting and should only be used with advice from an anesthetist.

Pump Implantation

Following successful screening, patients are encouraged to make an informed decision about whether to proceed to pump implantation. It is important to consider the cosmetic and practical effects of pump placement before surgery. Using a model pump, the individual and his partners can be encouraged to envisage the effects of various placement sites.

The surgical procedure ranges from 30 minutes to 2 hours, depending on the surgeon. The pump reservoir is filled during the operation, and intrathecal treatment can be commenced as soon as the patient is awake from the anesthetic. Often individuals want to titrate the intrathecal dose quickly, especially if they are keen to reduce their oral drugs. It is imperative that there is a clear titration plan, which allows multidisciplinary evaluation of effect over time. The majority of this work is done most effectively in the community setting. Slow intrathecal titration and oral baclofen reduction promotes safety, but also allows for changes in spasticity be assessed when the person is at home immersed again in his daily life. Dose titrations can then be tailored to his actual needs, rather than to perceived needs in the false hospital setting (73).

Complications

Apart from the usual surgical complications, mechanical problems sometimes occur. These can include catheter displacement or kinking, in which the catheter becomes stretched or is not properly anchored in place. The manufacturers suggest that a 1 to 2 cm loop of catheter should be left to accommodate any severe postoperative spasm that might stretch and disconnect the tubing. Pump displacement can sometimes occur in overweight people or those who gain considerable weight following pump implantation (74). This may require surgical review to resite the pump, but patients should be educated to prevent weight gain whenever possible. The pumps themselves are extremely reliable and incorporate a number of safety features, such as low-reservoir battery alarms and bacterioretentive filters. If a problem is suspected, specialist input may be required to enable safe detection of the cause. Protocols for troubleshooting problems, magnetic resonance imaging (MRI) surveillance, and use of radiopaque dye studies are required in specialist centers (73).

Some medical complications have been reported following the introduction of ITB. These can include excessive weakness, headache, drowsiness, respiratory depression, and pyrexia within the first 48 hours (70). When limbs become flaccid, venous return can be compromised, leading to deep vein thromboses and pulmonary embolism (76). Other reported complications include orthostatic hypotension, loss of penile erections, postsurgical meningocele, and generalized seizures associated with rapid withdrawal of the drug (77). Urinary output should be monitored postoperatively, because retention of urine can occur. However, improvements in bladder dysfunction have been reported as long-term benefits in some studies (78,79).

Patient Education

Intrathecal baclofen treatment requires the patient to take an active role in negotiating ongoing management. It is therefore important that factual information on which to base these decisions be available at each stage in the process. The nurse, in collaboration with the physical therapist and doctor, helps the patient identify achievable goals and realistic expectations of ITB therapy.

Psychological support is often need ed at all stages, including after the patient returns home. A well-coordinated service provides effective liaison and education for community healthcare professionals, as well as for patients and caregivers. It is also important to provide a strategy for responding to emergency queries at any time. The patient's knowledge should be consolidated by written instructions on ITB therapy and emergency safety measures, including contact numbers for 24–hour advice and information. He should also be aware of the role of noxious stimuli in exacerbating spasticity and how to prevent such situations from occurring whenever possible. A pump identification card is provided with each Medtronic pump. This details the serial number of the pump, what drug it contains, and the contact details of its refill center. The patient should be encouraged to carry this at all times in case of emergency and especially if needing to pass through any security cordons, such as at airports.

Follow-Up Management

Depending on the concentration and the rate of baclofen used, a patient usually will need to have the pump refilled every 3 to 4 months. In the United Kingdom, this is usually done at a specialist center, whereas in North America it is often done at home. Refilling involves introducing a needle through the skin into the access port of the pump, withdrawing the remaining solution, and refilling the reservoir with baclofen. The pump is reprogrammed and, at this point, it is possible to make fine adjustments to the dosage in response to the patient's reports of effectiveness and the healthcare professional's assessment.

An alarm indicates the need to replace the pump battery after 5 to 7 years. This requires complete replacement of the pump, although the catheter may be left in place if patent. It can be a good time to update the person about spasticity management and ITB therapy, because often the technology will have advanced.

It can be seen that this high-technology treatment for severe spasticity requires considerable organization and coordination of multidisciplinary input to provide an effective and safe form of management (3,75). A nurse-coordinated service provides a good model of care in this respect (73,74).

Intrathecal Phenol

Phenol (benzyl alcohol) is a neurolytic chemical that, when injected intrathecally, leads to cell damage, axonal degeneration, and indiscriminate destruction of motor and sensory nerves. Phenol will only have an effect on the neural component of tone and not on any biomechanical changes intrinsic to the muscles or soft tissues (73). It can be a useful treatment option in cases of severe lower limb spasticity, particularly in reducing pain, promoting improved postures, and increasing ease for caregivers. In one study, a reduction in adductor tone and spasms led to improved sexual function for two women (80).

Potential Side Effects

Short-term side effects may include hypotension, heart rate and rhythm disturbances secondary to sympathetic nerve blockade, and occasionally respiratory depression, occurring during or in the immediate postinjection period. Post-procedure the individual may experience a low-pressure headache secondary to CSF leakage.

Long-term side effects can include changes in muscle power and sensation, and in sexual, bowel, and bladder function. In addition to sensory impairment causing numbness, some patients may experience a change in sensation, with the appearance of dysesthetic pain or alteration in the character of pre-existing pain.

Patient Selection

Careful patient selection is required to minimize the impact of long-term side effects (80–82) . The use of intrathecal phenol should only be considered when other spasticity management strategies become ineffective. Criteria that may suggest intrathecal phenol is appropriate to consider include (a) the presence of marked motor loss, (b) reduced sensation of the lower limbs, and (c) significant, but effectively managed bladder and bowel dysfunction perhaps through the use of suprapubic catheters or regular enemas (73).

The Treatment Procedure

Phenol treatment involves two phases: the trial and the injection. Considerable expertise is required, not only because it is a destructive treatment but because the procedure is technically difficult due to the restricted position the person can be placed in to disperse the phenol, both during and after the procedure.

The trial phase involves injecting a short-acting anesthetic agent such as bupivacaine into the intrathecal space. The trial allows the patient to temporarily experience the effect of the phenol injection and forms an important part of the education process. Experiencing the injection, especially for individuals with cognitive impairment, can often help consolidate verbal and written information and show how the injection may affect their daily life (73). If the trial injection is successful, and the person wishes to go ahead, the process of giving the phenol injection can be arranged and is similar to the trial procedure. Medical and nursing procedures for this treatment have recently been detailed (73). The effects of intrathecal phenol can diminish over time, and repeat injections maybe required. Liaison with the person's community team is paramount to ensure ongoing care and to identify when any further input maybe needed (73). Its impacton spasticity and positioning can be dramatic, so it is likely the individual will need a seating review to prevent complications and accommodate this sudden change in posture. For these reasons, it is imperative that intrathecal phenol treatment is carried out in close liaison with the relevant seating specialists, physiotherapists, or occupational therapists.

Although the destructiveness of intrathecal phenol as a treatment option necessitates careful patient selection, for the small group who are suitable, it can have a dramatic impact on reducing spasticity and spasms and promoting their comfort, ease of care, and quality of life.

Surgical Interventions

The surgical procedures of anterior or posterior rhizotomy have been used for many years with varying degrees of success. The fact that these procedures are destructive and irreversible limits their use in clinical practice. However, modern microsurgical techniques mean that more selective procedures are now available. Modern techniques include microsurgical lesions of the dorsal root entry zone (DREZ) of the lateral roots, resulting in the destruction of small nociceptive afferents with the preservation of large fibers. A less invasive technique is the application of percutaneous radiofrequency rhizotomy, which has been reported to decrease spasticity with minimal risk to sexual or sphincter function (83). These techniques are highly specialized and currently are rarely applied. Their use is limited to patients for whom all other forms of treatment have been considered or have failed.

Summary

Spasticity is a common symptom of MS, and one that has far-reaching effects on many aspects of daily life for those affected. Despite the fact that its exact pathophysiology is still poorly understood, a wide range of treatment and management options have been developed that can alleviate existing spasticity and help prevent the development of associated complications. These options call on the skills of a range of healthcare professionals who need to work together in partnership with the patient and his family if effective outcomes are to be achieved.

In general, simple noninvasive therapies should be tried before resorting to more complex forms of management. In all cases, the person with MS and his family must be actively involved and become knowledgeable partners with healthcare professionals to jointly manage the problem. As a result of their holistic approach, organizational skills, and close patient relationships, specialist nurses are able to provide much-needed advice, education, treatment, and coordination in this complex area of management.

REFERENCES

1. Rizzo MA, Hadjimichael OC, Preiningerova J, Vollmer TL. Prevalence and treatment of spasticity reported by multiple sclerosis patients. *Multiple Sclerosis.* 2004;10:589–595.
2. Thompson AJ, Jarrett L, Lockley L, et al. Clinical management of spasticity. Editorial. *J Neurol Neurosurg Psychiatry.* 2005;76:459–463.
3. Stevenson VL, Jarrett L, eds. *Spasticity Management: A Practical Multidisciplinary Guide.* Oxford: Taylor & Francis, 2006.

4. Jarrett L. Provision of education and promoting self-management. In: Stevenson V, Jarrett L, eds. *Spasticity Management: A Practical Multidisciplinary Guide*. Oxford: Taylor & Francis, 2006.

5. Lance JW. Symposium synopsis. In: Feldman RG, Young RR, Koella WP, eds. *Spasticity: Disordered Motor Control*. Chicago: Year Book Medical Publishers; 1980:485–494.

6. Pandyan AD, Gregoric M, Barnes MP, et al. Spasticity: Clinical perceptions, neurological realities and meaningful measurement. *Disability Rehab*. 2005;27(1/2):2–6.

7. Sheean G. Neurophysiology of spasticity. In: Barnes MP, Johnson GR. *Upper Motor Neurone Syndrome and Spasticity: Clinical Management and Neurophysiology*. New York: Cambridge University Press, 2001.

8. Stevenson VL, Marsden JF. What is spasticity? In: Stevenson V, Jarrett L, eds. *Spasticity Management: A Practical Multidisciplinary Guide*. Oxford: Taylor & Francis, 2006.

9. Carr J, Shepherd R. *Neurological Rehabilitation: Optimising Motor Performance*. Oxford: Butterworth-Heinemann, 1998.

10. Sharkey FC. Medical and surgical management of spasticity. *Clin Neurosurg*. 1980;28: 589–596.

11. Losseff N, Thompson AJ. The medical management of increased tone. *Physiotherapy*. 1995;81(8):480–484.

12. Porter B. Nursing management of spasticity. *Primary Healthcare*. 2001;11(1):25–29.

13. Currie R. Spasticity: A common symptom of multiple sclerosis. *Nurs Stand*. 2001;15(33):47–52.

14. Jarrett L. The role of the nurse in the management of spasticity. *Nurs Residential Care*. 2004;6(3):116–119.

15. Holland NJ, Stockwell S. Controlling spasticity (patient pamphlet). New York: National Multiple Sclerosis Society, 1998.

16. Richardson D. Evaluation of interventions in the management of spasticity: Treatment goals and outcome measures. In: Sheean G, Barnes MP, eds. *Spasticity Rehabilitation*. London: Churchill Communications Europe; 1998:57–69.

17. Platz T, Eickhof C, Nuyens G, Vuadens P. Clinical scales for the assessment of spasticity, associated phenomena, and function: a systematic review of the literature. *Disability Rehab*. 2005;27(1/2):7–18.

18. Wood DE, Burridge JH, Van Wijck F, et al. Biomenchanical approaches applied to the lower and upper limb for the measurement of spasticity: A systematic review of the literature. *Disability Rehab*. 2005;27(1/2):19–32.

19. Voerman GE, Gregoric M, Hermens HJ. Neurophysiological methods for the assessment of spasticity: The Hoffman reflex, the tendon reflex, and the stretch reflex. *Disability Rehab*. 2005;27(1/2):33–68.

20. Hobart J, Riazi A, Thompson A, et al. Getting the measure of spasticity in MS: The Multiple Sclerosis Society Spasticity Scale (MSSS-88). *Brain*. 2006; in press.

21. Ashworth B. Preliminary trial of carisoprodol in multiple sclerosis. *Practitioner*. 1964;192:540–542.

22. Penn RD, Savoy SM, Corcos D, et al. Intrathecal baclofen for severe spinal spasticity. *N Engl J Med*. 1989;320(23):1517–1521.

23. Charmaz K. Loss of self: A fundamental form of suffering in the chronically ill. *Sociology Health Illness*. 1983;5(2):168–195.

24. Kralik D. The quest for ordinariness: Transition experienced by midlife woman living with chronic illness. *J Advanced Nurs*. 2002;39(2):1146–1154.

25. Lockley L, Buchanan K. Physical management of spasticity. In: Stevenson V, Jarrett L, eds. *Spasticity Management: A Practical Multidisciplinary Guide*. Oxford: Taylor & Francis, 2006.

26. O'Connell E. Exercise therapy in multiple sclerosis. *Physiother Ireland*. 2005;26:23–26.

27. Rietberg M, Brooks D, Uitdehaag B, Kwakkel G. Exercise therapy for multiple sclerosis. *Cochrane Database Syst Rev*. 2004;3:CD003980.

28. Brown P. Pathophysiology of spasticity. *J Neurol Neurosurg Psychiatry*. 1994;57:773–777.

29. Edwards S. Analysis of normal movement. In: Edwards S, ed. *Neurological Physiotherapy: A Problem Solving Approach*. London: Churchill Livingstone; 1996:15–20.

30. Edwards S. Physiotherapy management of established spasticity. In: Sheean G, Barnes MP, eds. *Spasticity Rehabilitation*. London: Churchill Communications Europe; 1998:71–89.

31. Pope P. Postural management and special seating. In: Edwards S, ed. *Neurological Physiotherapy: A Problem-Solving Approach*. London: Churchill Livingstone; 1996:135–160.

32. Barnes M, McLelland L, Sutton R. Spasticity. In: Greenwood R, Barnes MP, McMillan TM, et al., eds. *Neurological Rehabilitation*. London: Churchill Livingstone, 1993.

33. Johnson J. What can specialist nurses offer in caring for people with multiple sclerosis? In: Thompson AJ, Polman C, Hohlfeld R, eds. *Multiple Sclerosis: Clinical Challenges and Controversies*. London: Martin Dunitz; 1997:335–343.

34. Gracies JM, Nance P, Elovic E, et al. Traditional pharmacological treatments for spasticity. Part 2: General and regional treatments. *Muscle Nerve*. 1997;6(Suppl):S92–S120.

35. Shakespeare DT, Boggild M, Young C. Anti-spasticity agents for multiple sclerosis. *Cochrane Database Syst Rev*. 2003;4:CD001332.

36. Beard S, Hunn A, Wight J. Treatments for spasticity and pain in multiple sclerosis: A systematic review. *Health Technol Assess*. 2003;7(40):iii, ix–x, 1–111.

37. Paisley S, Beard S, Hunn A, Wight J. Clinical effectiveness of oral treatments for spasticity in multiple sclerosis: A systematic review. *Multiple Sclerosis*. 2002;8:319–329.

38. Cartlidge NE, Hudgson P, Weightman D. A comparison of baclofen and diazepam in the treatment of spasticity. *J Neurol Sci*. 1974;23:17–24.

39. From A, Heltberg A. A double-blind trial with baclofen (Lioresal) and diazepam in spasticity due to multiple sclerosis. *Acta Neurol Scand*. 1975;51:158–166.

40. Roussan M, Terence C, Fromm G. Baclofen versus diazepam for the treatment of spasticity and long-term follow-up of baclofen therapy. *Pharmatherapeutica*. 1985;5:278–284.

41. Emre M, Leslie GC, Muir C, et al. Correlations between dose, plasma concentrations, and antispastic action of tizanidine. *J Neurol Neurosurg Psychiatry*. 1994;57:1355–1359.

42. UK Tizanidine Trial Group, 1994.

43. Stevenson VL. Oral medication. In: Stevenson V, Jarrett L, eds. *Spasticity Management: A Practical Multidisciplinary Guide*. Oxford: Taylor & Francis, 2006.

44. Mueller ME, Gruenthal M, Olson WL, Olson WH. Gabapentin for relief of upper motor neuron symptoms in multiple sclerosis. *Arch Phys Med Rehabil*. 1997;78(5):521–524.

45. Cutter NC, Scott DD, Johnson JC, Whiteneck G. Gabapentin effect on spasticity in multiple sclerosis: A placebo-controlled, randomized trial. *Arch Phys Med Rehabil.* 2000;81(2): 164–169.

46. Howlett AC, Barth F, Bonner TI, et al. International union of pharmacology: XXVII, classification of cannabinoid receptors. *Pharmacol Rev.* 2002;54:161–202.

47. Wade DT, Robson P, House H, et al. A preliminary controlled study to determine whether whole-plant cannabis extracts can improve intractable neurogenic symptoms. *Clin Rehabil.* 2003;17:21–29.

48. Wade DT, Makela P, Robson P, et al. Do cannabis-based medicinal extracts have general or specific effects on symptoms in multiple sclerosis? A double-blind, randomized, placebo-controlled study on 160 patients. *Clin Rehabil.* 2004;10:434–441.

49. Zajicek J, Fox P, Sanders H, et al. Cannabinoids for treatment of spasticity and other symptoms related to multiple sclerosis (CAMS study): Multicentre randomised placebo-controlled trial. *Lancet.* 2003;362:1517–1526.

50. Fox P, Bain PG, Glickman S, et al. The effect of cannabis on tremor in patients with multiple sclerosis. *Neurology.* 2004;62:1105–1109.

51. Vaney C, Heinzel-Gutenbrunner M, Jobin P, et al. Efficacy, safety and tolerability of an orally administered cannabis extract in the treatment of spasticity in patients with multiple sclerosis: A randomized, double-blind, placebo-controlled, crossover study. *Multiple Sclerosis.* 2004;10:417–442.

52. Brady CM, DasGupta R, Dalton C, et al. An open-label pilot study of cannabis-based extracts for bladder dysfunction in advanced multiple sclerosis. *Multiple Sclerosis.* 2004;10:425–433.

53. Zajicek JP, Sanders HP, Wright DE, et al. Cannabinoids in multiple sclerosis (CAMS) study: Safety and efficacy data for 12 months follow-up. *J Neurol Neurosurg Psychiatry.* 2005;76:1664–1669.

54. Rao SM, Leo GJ, Bernadin L. Cognitive dysfunction in multiple sclerosis (i) frequency, patterns, prediction. *Neurology.* 1991;41:685–691.

55. Sadovnick AD, Remick RA, Allen J, et al. Depression in multiple sclerosis. *Neurology.* 1996;46:628–632.

56. van Kuijk AA, Geurts AC, et al. Treatment of upper extremity spasticity in stroke patients by focal neuronal or neuromuscular blockade: A systematic review of the literature. *J Rehab Med.* 2002;34(2):51–61.

57. Hesse S, Jahnke MT, et al. Short-term electrical stimulation enhances the effectiveness of Botulinum toxin in the treatment of lower limb spasticity in hemiparetic patients. *Neurosci Lett.* 1995;201(1):37–40.

58. Bhakta BB, Cozens JA, et al. Use of botulinum toxin in stroke patients with severe upper limb spasticity. *J Neurol Neurosurg Psychiatry.* 1996;61(1):30–35.

59. Simpson DM, Alexander DN, et al. Botulinum toxin type A in the treatment of upper extremity spasticity: A randomized, double-blind, placebo-controlled trial. *Neurology.* 1996;46(5):1306–1310.

60. Richardson DS, Edwards S, et al. The effect of botulinum toxin on hand function after incomplete spinal cord injury at the level of C5/6: A case report. *Clin Rehab.* 1997;11(4):288–292.

61. Bhakta BB, Cozens JA, et al. Impact of botulinum toxin type A on disability and carer burden due to arm spasticity after stroke: A randomised double blind placebo controlled trial. [erratum appears in *J Neurol Neurosurg Psychiatry* 2001;70(6):821.] *J Neurol Neurosurg Psychiatry.* 2000;69(2):217–221.

62. Rodriquez AA, McGinn M, et al. Botulinum toxin injection of spastic finger flexors in hemiplegic patients. *Am J Physical Med Rehab.* 2000;79(1):44–47.

63. Smith SJ, Ellis E, et al. A double-blind placebo-controlled study of botulinum toxin in upper limbspasticity after stroke or head injury. *Clin Rehab.* 2000;14(1):5–13.

64. Bakheit AM, Sawyer J. The effects of botulinum toxin treatment on associated reactions of the upper limb on hemiplegic gait: A pilot study. *Disability Rehab.* 2002;24(10):519–522.

65. Brashear A, Gordon MF, et al. Intramuscular injection of botulinum toxin for the treatment of wrist and finger spasticity after a stroke. [Comment.] *N Engl J Med.* 2002;347(6): 395–400.

66. RCP, Royal College of Physicians. Guidelines for the use of botulinum toxin (BTX) in the management of spasticity in adults. Clinical Effectiveness and Evaluation Unit, 2002.

67. Sheean GL. Botulinum treatment of spasticity: Why is it difficult to show a functional benefit? *Trauma Rehab.* 2001;771–776.

68. Mattison PG. TENS in the management of painful muscle spasm in patients with MS. *Clin Rehab.* 1993;7:45–48.

69. Penn RD, Kroin JS. Intrathecal baclofen alleviates spinal cord spasticity. *Lancet.* 1984;I:1078.

70. Jarrett L, Leary SM, Porter B, et al. Managing spasticity in people with multiple sclerosis. A goal orientated approach to intrathecal baclofen therapy. *Intern J MS Care.* 2001;3:2–11.

71. Price GW, Wilking GP, Turnball MJ, Bowery NG. Are baclofen-sensitive GABA$_A$ receptors present on primary afferent terminals of the spinal cord? *Nature.* 1984;307:71–74.

72. Lazorthes Y, Sallerin-Caule B, Verdie JC, et al. Chronic intrathecal baclofen administration for control of severe spasticity. *J Neurosurg.* 1990;72:393–402.

73. Jarrett L. Intrathecal therapies including baclofen and phenol. 8. Stevenson VL, Marsden JF. What is spasticity? In: Stevenson V, Jarrett L, eds. *Spasticity Management: A Practical Multidisciplinary Guide.* Oxford: Taylor & Francis, 2006.

74. Porter B. A review of intrathecal baclofen in the management of spasticity. *Br J Nurs.* 1997;6(5):253–262.

75. Becker WJ, Harris CJ, Long MI, et al. Long-term intrathecal baclofen therapy in patients with intractable spasticity. *Can J Neurol Sci.* 1995;22:208–217.

76. Zierski J, Muller H, Dralle D, Wurdinger T. Implanted pump systems for treatment of spasticity. *Acta Neurochir Suppl* (Wien). 1988;43:94–99.

77. Meythaler Steers WD, Tuel SM, Cross LL, Haworth CS. Continuous intrathecal baclofen in spinal cord spasticity: A prospective study. *Am J Phys Med Rehabil.* 1992;71:6:321–327.

78. Frost F, Nanninga JB, Penn RD, et al. Intrathecal baclofen infusion: Effects on bladder management programmes in patients with myelopathy. *Am J Phys Med Rehabil.* 1989;68(3): 112–115.

79. Nanninga JB, Frost F, Penn RD. Effects of intrathecal baclofen on bladder and sphincter function. *J Urol.* 1989;142(2):101–105.

80. Jarrett L, Nandi P, Thompson AJ. Managing severe lower limb spasticity in multiple sclerosis: Does intrathecal phenol have a role? *J Neurol Neurosurg Psychiatry.* 2002;73(6):705–709.

81. Werring D, Thompson AJ. Medical and surgical treatment of spasticity. In: Sheean G, Barnes MP, eds. *Spasticity Rehabilitation*. London: Churchill Communications Europe; 1998:92–107.

82. Williams JE, Shepherd J, Williams K. Rediscovery of an old technique to treat severe spasticity: intrathecal phenol. *Br J Therapy Rehab*. 1995;2(4):209–210.

83. Kadson DL, Lathi ES. A prospective study of radiofrequency rhizotomy in the treatment of post-traumatic spasticity. *Neurosurgery*. 1984;15:526–529.

CHAPTER 13

Pulmonary Complications

Linda Lehman, Mary Ann Picone, and June Halper

Pulmonary dysfunction secondary to multiple sclerosis (MS) is a leading cause of morbidity and mortality in this patient population who have advanced or worsening disease. Despite the fact that many emergency room and intensive care unit admissions are attributed to infectious and aspiration pneumonias leading to atelectasis and eventual respiratory failure, no protocols exist for evaluating and managing pulmonary dysfunction in MS. Publications on symptom management in MS deal with such symptoms as spasticity, bowel and bladder dysfunction, impaired cognition, visual disturbances, and dysphagia, but they fail to address the signs and symptoms of hypoventilation—dyspnea, orthopnea, weak cough, hypophonia, and fatigue. Fatigue is generally assumed to be the overwhelming lassitude peculiar to MS and not necessarily secondary to pulmonary dysfunction. A proposed protocol to be used in the management of pulmonary dysfunction in MS draws heavily on the practice of John R. Bach, M.D., and his associates, who have treated patients with a variety of neuromuscular diseases, including muscular dystrophy, amyotrophic lateral sclerosis, and spinal muscular atrophy (Figure 13-1) (1). Treatment is predicated on noninvasive interventions, the goals of which are to (a) prevent respiratory failure by maintaining normal lung ventilation, (b) maintain normal lung compliance, and (c) help eliminate airway secretions through more effective cough flows (1).

BERNARD W. GIMBEL

MULTIPLE SCLEROSIS
COMPREHENSIVE CARE CENTER
AT HOLY NAME HOSPITAL

718 TEANECK ROAD
TEANECK, NJ 07666
(201) 837-0727
(201) 837-8504 FAX

Gimbel MS Center
Pulmonary Assessment

Patient Name:	Date	Date	Date
HX of hospitalizations for respiratory infection			
Shortness of breath			
Recent respiratory infection			
Orthopnea			
Hypophonia			
Dysphagia			
VC Sitting			
VC Supine			
SaO_2			
$ETCO_2$			
Peak Cough Flow Assisted			
Peak Cough Flow Unassisted			
Nurses Initials			
Comments			

FIGURE 13-1

Five case studies are used to illustrate how these interventions have been used to maintain patients in the community and avoid long-term institutionalization.

Pathophysiology

Ventilation is the movement of air into and out of the lungs. The mechanics of ventilation follow Boyle's law of physics, which states that the pressure of gases is in direct proportion to the volume of the container. Gases move from an area of high pressure to one of lower pressure to maintain equilibrium (2).

The principal muscle of respiration is the dome-shaped diaphragm, which lies below the lungs. During inspiration, the diaphragm flattens, forcing the abdomen downward and expanding the chest cavity. This causes an increase in the thoracic volume, which leads thoracic pressure to fall below atmospheric pressure. As a result, air enters the lungs to fill the chest cavity. During expiration, the diaphragm relaxes, causing a decrease in thoracic volume and an increase in thoracic pressure. Air is then forced out of the lungs to stabilize the pressure (2).

The muscles of respiration include not only the diaphragm but also the external intercostal muscles and the accessory muscles (scalene and sternocleido-mastoid). The diaphragm is innervated by the phrenic nerve and the nerves at C3–C5. Paralysis of the diaphragm causes a paradoxical movement of the diaphragm upward, not downward, during inspiration (2).

The external intercostal muscles are innervated by the nerves of the thoracic spine. Contraction of these muscles causes the ribs to rise and rotate, a movement that pushes the sternum forward, enlarging the chest from front to back. Paralysis of the external intercostal muscles does not seriously affect respiration so long as the diaphragm is unaffected (2).

The scalene muscle raises the first and second ribs during inspiration, whereas the sternocleidomastoid raises the sternum. Neither muscle contributes significantly to quiet breathing, but they both play a key role during heavy exercise.

In contrast to inspiration, which requires the active contraction of muscles, expiration is generally a passive event during which the muscles of respiration relax and the lungs elastically recoil. However, during forced expiration, the abdominal and internal intercostal muscles are used for assistance.

The function of respiration is under the neurologic control of the medulla and pons. This region of the brain also gives rise to the cranial nerves that play a key role in the mechanics of chewing, movement of the tongue, and swallowing (cranial nerves V, VII, IX, X, XI, and XII). Injury to the pons and medulla therefore affects not only respiration but also the motor function of chewing and swallowing. Multiple sclerosis patients with lesions in this area are especially prone to aspiration of food and liquid, which predisposes them to aspiration pneumonias.

Respiration is essentially an involuntary action, although some respiratory movements such as sighing, speaking, laughing, and crying are under the voluntary control of the cerebral cortex. The impulse to breathe is triggered by chemore-ceptors that are sensitive to increased levels of carbon dioxide in the blood. These receptors send a message to the medulla, which in turn sends impulses to the muscles of respiration. Air enters the body through the nares and passes through the trachea, which bifurcates into the bronchi before subdividing into bronchioles. Within the lungs, gas exchange with the blood takes place in air sacs called *alveoli*. Oxygen diffuses from the alveoli into the blood, while carbon dioxide diffuses from the blood into the alveoli and is expelled from the body through exhaled air.

In MS, neuromuscular weakness leads to poor ventilation of the lung. As the muscles of inspiration weaken, the patient takes shallower breaths. A build-up of carbon dioxide in the blood occurs, which eventually rises above the norm of 35 to 44 mm Hg and leads to hypercapnia. Oxygen saturations fall below 95%, and the patient becomes hypoxic. Furthermore, as the muscles of expiration weaken, the patient is no longer able to cough effectively to clear secretions and is at high risk for atelectasis and pneumonia (1).

Studies of MS patients have identified the existence of pulmonary dysfunction and suggest that the problem may exist early in the disease process, before the patient becomes symptomatic. Smeltzer and coworkers (3) studied 25 MS patients with no apparent respiratory symptoms. Of those, ten were ambulatory with and without aids, seven were wheelchair-dependent, and eight were bedridden. Forced vital capacity, maximal voluntary ventilation, and maximal expiratory pressure were found to be below predicted values in bedridden and nonambulatory patients with upper extremity involvement. More recently, Grasso and colleagues (4) measured these values in 71 patients with secondary-progressive (SPMS) and primary-progressive MS (PPMS) and found that, although 63.4% of all subjects had abnormal values, there was greater incidence with nonambulatory patients (82.8%) than ambulatory patients (35.7%). Dysfunction also was positively correlated with the presence of cerebellar signs.

These studies suggest that MS patients should be evaluated for pulmonary dysfunction on a routine basis. Bach recommends evaluation at a minimum of every 6 to 12 months, but possibly every 1 to 3 months if rapid disease progression occurs (1).

Pulmonary Assessment

Equipment needs for evaluation are simple and inexpensive. Expensive pulmonary function tests and painful arterial blood gases are not necessary because these patients do not have underlying pulmonary disease. They have impairment of ventilation, not impaired oxygenation, as in chronic obstructive pulmonary disease (COPD). Likewise, polysomnography is not warranted because it cannot determine impaired ventilation secondary to neuromuscular weakness. Recommended equipment is as follows (1):

- Hand-held spirometer
- Pulse oximeter
- Peak flow meter
- Capnograph to measure end tidal CO_2

Important measurements to obtain are:

- Vital capacity (supine)
- Vital capacity (sitting)
- SaO_2
- $ETCO_2$
- Assisted cough flow
- Unassisted cough flow

Patients are also assessed for symptoms of chronic alveolar hypoventilation. This pulmonary assessment flowsheet is being adapted by our center for routine screening of nonambulatory patients.

The assessment of pulmonary dysfunction calls for interdisciplinary teamwork that includes the physician, nurse, and respiratory therapist. Assessment is needed for symptomatic patients and those with supine vital capacities less than sitting vital capacities, daytime SaO_2 less than 95%, and $ETCO_2$ greater than 44 mm Hg. These patients undergo nocturnal SaO_2 monitoring. If the patient has ten or more sawtooth oxyhemoglobin desaturations equal to or greater than 3% per hour and mean SaO_2 less than 94%, she is furnished with a bi-level positive airway pressure (BiPAP) machine (Respironics Inc., Murrysville, PA) for nocturnal nasal use (5).

BiPAP is a noninvasive inspiratory aid that assists in ventilating the patient with neuromuscular disease and reversing hypercapnia. It is far more effective than supplemental oxygen, which merely masks the hypoxia and can lead to hypercapnia by reducing the ventilatory drive so that the patient runs the risk of not breathing altogether (CO_2 narcosis) (6).

BiPAP delivers air continuously under positive pressure. The setting for delivery during inspiration is independent of that delivered during expiration. The difference between the inspiratory positive airway pressure (IPAP) and the expiratory positive airway pressure (EPAP) is known as the span. The greater the span, the greater the assistance in inspiratory effort. Current models of BiPAP have IPAPs of 20 to 30 cm H_2O. Low spans are inadequate for ventilation, reducing hypophonia, and maintaining lung compliance. A span of 18 to 25 cm H_2O is the minimum required to ventilate a normal lung. Although EPAP cannot be eliminated from BiPAP, it is set to a minimum of 2 to 3 cm H_2O. EPAP is more appropriate when there is evidence of obstructive sleep apnea, and it is not necessary to ventilate a patient with neuromuscular disease. As lung compliance diminishes, patients may need to be switched from BiPAP to a portable volume ventilator (1).

BiPAP and portable volume ventilators are noninvasive means of maintaining normal lung ventilation. They also help to maintain lung compliance by helping to maximize insufflation capacity. When respiratory muscles become weak, and patients are unable to inhale deeply, the lungs become stiff and prone to atelectasis. It is therefore important that patients engage in pulmonary range of motion (ROM) to maintain the elasticity of their lungs. Incentive spirometers are contraindicated because neuromuscular weakness impedes deep inhalations for active ROM. However, passive ROM can be accomplished with deep insufflations by air stacking with an Ambu bag or portable volume ventilator. The former requires the assistance of a caregiver. Pulmonary ROM should be initiated as soon as vital capacity reaches 50% to 60% of normal value, and should be performed no less than three times daily (1). We recommend that our patients keep a hand-held mouthpiece on their BiPAP machines or ventilators close to their chairs, and that they use it to take deep insufflations throughout the day for ROM of their respiratory muscles.

Cough flows should also be evaluated on an ongoing basis. A normal cough flow is 6 L/second with variations based on age, sex, and height. When values fall to 2.7 L/second or less, a cough is too weak to clear airway secretions without assistance. At this point, many patients with neuromuscular disease are inappropriately treated with bronchodilators and chest physical therapy (PT) and percussion. However, these interventions are ineffective because of the absence of underlying pulmonary disease. Cough flows can be increased by insufflating the lungs to maximum capacity and following this by a manual abdominal thrust given by a caregiver. When assisted cough flow falls below 2.7 L/second, especially during acute respiratory tract infection, the patient is at highest risk for respiratory failure because of inability to clear secretions (1,7).

Mechanical insufflation-exsufflation (MI-E) has eliminated the need for tracheostomy, bronchoscopy, and intubation during acute illness. By delivering deep, forceful inhalations at 30 to 50 cm H_2O, followed by immediate application of negative pressure of 30 to 50 cm H_2O for 1 to 3 seconds (exsufflation), accompanied by manual abdominal thrusts, patients with neuromuscular involvement of respiratory function are able to clear their airways. Protocol calls for 4 to 5 cycles of MI-E followed by independent breathing for 20 to 30 seconds to prevent hyperventilation. Cycles are repeated until secretions are cleared and SaO_2 returns to normal. During times of acute respiratory illness, patients may need to use the MI-E every 10 minutes over a 24-hour period (1,8,9).

The device now used for MI-E is the In-Exsufflator (JH Emerson Co., Cambridge, MA), which was approved by the U.S. Food and Drug Administration in 1993. The In-Exsufflator is well tolerated and shows no evidence of damaging side effects, including pneumothorax, hemoptysis, or aspiration of gastric contents (9).

Other Wellness Measures

In addition, it is imperative to recognize the role of rehabilitation related to this problem in terms of the importance of good body alignment while the patient is seated or reclining, individualized wheelchair prescriptions, and the appropriate assistive devices for safe ambulation and the promotion of full chest expansion. Other wellness measures to prevent secondary infections that might lead to pulmonary complications in MS include preventative immunizations (influenza vaccine, pneumonia vaccine) and prevention of skin breakdown that may result in prolonged immobility.

Case Study 1

The following case study exemplifies a typical scenario in which an MS patient is brought to the emergency room in respiratory distress secondary to pneumonia. Maria is a 45-year-old woman who has had PPMS since 1985. The mother of two teenage children, she is totally dependent in terms of her activities of daily living but has been able to continue to live at home with the help of a dedicated and conscientious home health aide. The patient was brought to the emergency room by ambulance with complaints of dyspnea. X-ray confirmed the presence of lower lobe infiltrates bilaterally. Arterial blood gases showed pCO_2 of 72.8 and pO_2 of 52. She was admitted to the ICU and intubated. However, over the course of the following week, Maria developed atelectasis and underwent tracheostomy with inflated cuff. This rendered her unable to speak or swallow, and she was given a percutaneous endoscopic gastrostomy (PEG) tube for feeding. Her discharge plan called for transfer to long-term care facility because it was assumed that both tracheostomy and PEG tube feeding were permanent.

Maria was still in the hospital after 1 month, at which time an experienced physician was called in for consultation. He immediately deflated the cuff, and the patient was able to speak, which suggested to him that bulbar function was still intact. SaO_2 at room air was 96% to 97%. It was agreed that Maria would be transferred to his service for removal of tracheostomy tube and initiation of noninvasive intermittent positive pressure ventilation (IPPV). This was accomplished within a week, and she was subsequently discharged home with a portable volume ventilator and In-Exsufflator.

Case Study 2

Carol is a 38-year-old woman with SPMS and asthma, for which she receives Flovent, Serevent, theophylline, and nebulized albuterol as needed. She also receives oxygen at 2 liters, as prescribed by her pulmonologist. She was diagnosed with MS in 1997, and has remained neurologically stable on subcutaneous (SC) Copaxone 20 mg daily. Carol is a former nurse manager now on long-term disability and currently living with her supportive husband and school-age child.

When first seen, Carol presented with dyspnea with minimal exertion, hypophonia, extreme fatigue, severe coughing, and headache. She reported that she choked on thin liquids. She also reported difficulty sleeping at night, with frequent arousals from sleep and the need to sleep on three pillows. She was started on BiPAP 12/5 in October 1998 and pulse oximetry in the home. It was noted that she had oxygen desaturations when sleeping and walking, but that SaO_2 recovered after a bout of severe coughing, which was attributed to aspiration of upper airway secretions. The span of Carol's BiPAP was increased to 20/5 for nighttime use, and she was prescribed IPPV via mouthpiece during the day whenever SaO_2 fell to 94%.

Six months later Carol was following all these recommendations. She was noticeably less short of breath and had greater amplification of voice. There also was significant improvement in vital capacity both sitting and supine. However, she still wakes up with headache, and pulse oximetry shows desaturations to 90% at night despite supplemental oxygen. This underlies the fact that Carol has a problem with hypoventilation, not oxygenation. The respiratory therapist recommended that settings on the BiPAP be increased to 25/5 and that the patient obtain a lip seal with Velcro band to prevent leakage of air through her mouth. If these interventions fail to maintain SaO_2 above 94%, Carol may need to be upgraded to a portable volume ventilator.

Case Study 3

Amy is a 36-year-old woman who has had SPMS since 1994. She is a homemaker with three children, aged 5, 7, and 9, and is struggling to meet the needs of her family and manage her home. There are significant financial constraints on the family because Amy's husband has had an inconsistent work history, which also has had negative consequences on the continuity of medical insurance.

The patient's MS has been managed by SC Betaseron 1 mL every other day. Nevertheless, she has had several exacerbations that have required treatment with intravenous (IV) Solu-Medrol. Amy now uses a motorized scooter for maximal mobility. Approximately 2 years ago, she was diagnosed with esophageal dysmotility and was placed on a dysphagia diet consisting of only pureed foods. At about this time, she began to complain of shortness of breath, fatigue, interrupted sleep, and severe orthopnea.

She was breathless with speech and unable to speak in sentences without pausing for breath every few words.

Amy was first seen by a pulmonologist, who found that her pulmonary function tests and chest X-ray were within normal limits. He concluded that there was no underlying pulmonary disease and that shortness of breath was related to a weakened diaphragm secondary to MS. Amy was referred back to her neurologist, who arranged for a home evaluation by a respiratory therapist. She was prescribed BiPAP for nocturnal use. At her follow-up evaluation 3 months later, she reported improvement in shortness of breath. She was able to speak in complete and audible sentences without any apparent breathlessness. Unassisted peak cough flow was 350. Amy further reported fewer interruptions in sleep patterns, and stated that she can now sleep until at least 3:00 A.M. without waking.

Case Study 4

Mike is a 33-year-old man who has had PPMS since 1986. He is quadriplegic, totally nonverbal, and fed via PEG tube because of dysphagia. At this time, Mike is essentially bedridden. Despite his disabilities, Mike is managed at home and is cared for by loving family members, who refuse to consider nursing home placement.

This patient has had numerous hospital admissions for infectious and aspiration pneumonias. In January 1998, he was admitted for respiratory insufficiency secondary to aspiration pneumonia and inability to clear secretions. Consideration was given to tracheostomy for pulmonary toilet. However, the family was reluctant to resort to such invasive means as a permanent solution to clearing of airways. Preference was expressed for noninvasive interventions. The decision was made to try the In-Exsufflator.

Mike's family was trained in the use of the In-Exsufflator, and he was discharged home with the equipment. The In-Exsufflator has enabled the family to continue to care for this patient in their home and to prevent further deterioration and complication in his respiratory status.

Case Study 5

This last case demonstrates some adherence issues occasionally encountered when prescribing use of the BiPAP. Sarah is a 58-year-old woman who has had PPMS since 1981. Her symptoms include severe hypophonia, fatigue, dyspnea, and ineffective cough. Pulmonary function tests showed no evidence of upper airway obstruction. $ETCO_2$ was within normal limits, and SaO_2 was 97%. Maximal inspiratory and expiratory pressures were below predicted value, and she showed no response to bronchodilators. The pulmonologist concluded that Sarah had severe ventilatory deficit and referred her back to our center.

The neurologist referred this patient for home evaluation by a respiratory therapist, who performed a nighttime pulse oximetry study. This confirmed that Sarah had desaturations to 85% during her sleep. She was prescribed BiPAP for nocturnal use via a nasal piece, and the equipment was delivered to her home. Follow-up phone calls to this patient revealed that the equipment was not being used as prescribed. Sarah cited discomfort with the headpiece as the reason for nonuse of the BiPAP. The respiratory therapist made additional visits to her home to refit the headpiece, but Sarah was adamant in her refusal to attach the device to her head. A joint visit was made by the respiratory therapist and the nurse to assess barriers to adherence. At this visit, the respiratory therapist assembled the handheld mouthpiece of the BiPAP and secured it to the patient's wheelchair so that she could use it on an as-needed basis throughout the day and demonstrated to the patient the benefit of using this device to amplify her voice. Sarah has continued to use the BiPAP with the handheld piece during the daytime, but she still refuses to use the device at night. However, daytime use alone has improved her ability to talk on the phone and make conversation.

The Role of the Nurse

Nurses play an important role in the interdisciplinary team treating MS patients. The first assessment of the patient usually is by a nurse. It is important that MS nurses become sensitive to the problem of hypoventilation secondary to neuromuscular weakness and carefully screen the patient for symptoms of dyspnea, dysphagia, weak cough, sleep disturbance, and so forth. History taking should elicit information about recent and recurring respiratory tract infections. All patients at risk for hypoventilation should be referred for evaluation according to the preceding outlined protocol.

Nurses also play a major role in implementation of the plan and in adherence by the patient to the prescribed treatment. As the last case study clearly demonstrates, it is the nurse who assesses barriers to adherence and facilitates formulation of a revised plan. As educators, nurses reinforce to patient and caregiver the importance of following the plan of care. Finally, it is important to continuously follow-up with the patient and caregiver to assess continued benefit of treatment.

Conclusion

This small sample of patients suggests that noninvasive positive pressure ventilation, mechanical insufflation-exsufflation, and pulse oximetry can be used prophylactically to prevent respiratory complications in MS patients. Based on the few positive outcomes seen at our center, further study is proposed in which a large sample of patients will be followed-up longitudinally to assess continued benefit from noninvasive respiratory aids.

The protocol outlined promises to reduce the risk of hospitalization and highly invasive procedures such as intubation, tracheostomy, and bronchoscopy. A considerable advantage of employing noninvasive respiratory aids is that patients generally can be managed at home, thus avoiding the possibility of institutionalization in a long-term care facility. In addition, the noninvasive interventions are less costly than treating the patient for respiratory failure in an acute care facility, where they are more likely to undergo the high-tech and invasive procedures that normally accompany such stays. However, insurance companies do not routinely pay for preventive care, and healthcare professionals need to educate them about the sequelae of pulmonary dysfunction in neuromuscular diseases such as MS (9).

REFERENCES

1.　Bach JR. *Guide to the Evaluation and Management of Neuromuscular Disease.* Philadelphia: Hanley & Belfus, 1999.

2.　Porth CM. *Pathophysiology: Concepts of Altered Health States,* 3rd ed. Philadelphia: Lippincott, 1990.

3.　Smeltzer SC, Utell MJ, Rudick RA, Herndon RM. Pulmonary function and dysfunction in multiple sclerosis. *Arch Neurol.* 1988; 45:1245–1249.

4.　Grasso MG, Lubich S, Guidi L, et al. *Cerebellar deficit and respiratory impairment in patients with multiple sclerosis.* Paper presented at the Second World Congress in Neurological Rehabilitation, Toronto, Ontario, 1999.

5.　Bach JR. Non-invasive management and prevention of respiratory complications of multiple

CHAPTER 14

Pain

Heidi Maloni

Pain is a symptom experienced in three-quarters of people with multiple sclerosis (MS) at some time during the disease course. Pain may be a presenting symptom occurring at all levels of disability, typically affecting equally age, gender, and MS classification. The frequency and intensity of the pain experience in MS varies. Pain in MS is associated with anxiety, fatigue, and depression (1–7). Because the symptom of pain has such a pervasive impact on quality of life for people with MS who experience it, the caring nurse is challenged to make a difference. It is the aim of this chapter to give the advanced practice MS nurse the understanding and ability to meet the challenge and manage the life-altering effects of pain in patients with MS.

Pain is complex, difficult to define and quantify. The MS nurse recognizes that pain is a subjective sensory symptom: Pain is whatever the experiencing person says it is, existing whenever she says it does (8). The International Association for the Study of Pain (IASP), defines pain as an unpleasant sensory and emotional experience associated with actual or potential tissue damage, or described in terms of such damage. The IASP also states that pain is an individualistic, learned, and social response to an unpleasant or noxious stimuli (9). Several biologic events make up the experience of pain. Understanding the subjective nature, and the influence of learned and social response to pain assists the MS nurse in exploring varied approaches to its management in MS.

Pain Experience

The experience of pain is multidimensional, a culmination of physical, psychological, and social factors having sensory, emotional, and cognitive aspects. The experience of pain is truly a mind-body phenomenon, as evidenced by three systems that interact to produce and control pain experience. The *sensory/discriminative system* informs the person of the strength, intensity, and location of the sensation of pain. Pain sensations are mediated by afferent sensory fibers from spinal cord to cortex, resulting in actions such as instantaneous withdrawal from touching a hot stove. The function of the *motivational/affective system* is a determination of the individual's conditioned, learned, or emotional response to pain. Approach/avoidance behaviors are mediated through the reticular formation, the limbic system, and the brain stem. Examples include animal-level behaviors, instinctual protective behaviors of isolation, guarding, seeking shelter or protection, or emotional responses of fear and distress. The *cognitive/evaluative system* functions to determine the interpretation of the appropriate response to pain at the cortical level. Determinations are made on cultural preference, male and female roles, and past experience. The cognitive/evaluative system may block, modulate, or enhance the perception of pain. Examples include role, societal and cultural expectations, or cultural adages such as, "Big boys don't cry," "Offer it up," "Be mature," "No pain, no gain" (10).

No direct relationship exists between the intensity of painful stimuli and an individual's perception of or response to pain. The experience of pain is influenced by pain threshold and pain tolerance. Pain *threshold* is the point at which a stimulus is perceived as pain. The point of pain perception does not vary significantly from person to person or in the same individual over time. Threshold can vary when an individual experiences competing pain and a phenomenon of perceptual dominance is exhibited. The brain attends to one pain stimuli at a time based on intensity. Intense pain at one site may increase the pain threshold at another site. Alternately, when the dominant pain is reduced, the individual is cognizant of other painful areas (11). An example is the carpenter who cut off his hand with a band saw and responded to his hand pain by shooting nails from his nail gun into his skull. Neurologists suggested that the carpenter's hand pain was diminished by the pain suffered from the nail gun to his skull, because the brain was distracted from one injury and prioritized the second injury (12). It is also interesting to note that the carpenter was using the motivational/affective system to modulate his pain experience.

Pain tolerance is the duration of time or the intensity of pain that an individual will endure before initiating a response. Because an individual's physiological response to painful stimuli varies, pain tolerance also varies from person to person and can be different in the same person over time (11). A headache suffered all day finally brings the individual to the aspirin bottle in the evening. Reasons for not treating the headache sooner relate to tolerability. Pain tolerance is influenced by culture, role, expectation, and general physical and mental health. Tolerance to pain is decreased with repeated exposure to pain, stress, fatigue, anger, boredom, apprehension, and sleep deprivation. Pain tolerance is increased with alcohol consumption, medication, hypnosis, warmth, distracting activities, and strong beliefs or faith (8). Competing stimuli such as distraction, socialization, and recreation, may act to increase pain tolerance and raise the pain threshold. Understanding concepts such as the experience of pain, pain tolerance, pain threshold, and perceptual dominance creates rationale for the practice of MS pain management by the MS nurse.

Assessment

Assessment is the MS nurse's most powerful weapon in the war to effectively manage MS pain. During a thorough and guided assessment, nurse and patient establish a relationship based on mutual trust and respect. This foundation allows the patient and the nurse to engage in mutual goal setting that effectuates positive outcomes for the MS patient experiencing pain.

Adequate assessment of pain requires time and knowledge. Knowledge of pharmacologic management, side-effect management, and nonpharmacologic strategies to manage MS pain gives the nurse the confidence to guide treatment. Patients may be reluctant to discuss the symptom of pain because they have low expectations for pain relief. Patients may be unwilling to take multiple medications and unwilling to suffer the side effects of medications. Patients may feel their pain is less significant than bowel and bladder dysfunction or weakness. Stoicism, the "good patient" syndrome, communication skills, and cognitive ability may all become barriers to a complete pain assessment. Critical thinking skills on the part of the MS nurse are acquired through assessment.

The nursing assessment of pain is guided by the use of the mnemonic OLD CART:

+ **O**–*Onset*: When did your pain begin?
+ **L**–*Location*: Where is your pain?
+ **D**–*Duration*: How long does your pain last?
+ **C**–*Characteristics*: Describe your pain, what is it like, the severity, and the intensity.
+ **A**–*Aggravators*: What makes your pain worse?
+ **R**–*Relievers*: What relieves your pain?
+ **T**–*Treatment*: What are you using, doing, and taking to minimize the pain?

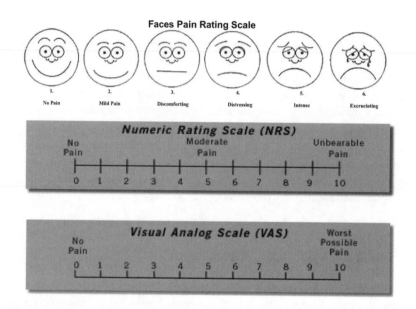

Self-report pain intensity measurement scales. Used with permission from Jacox A, et al., AHCPR, 1994; and Hockenberry MJ, Wilson D, Winkelstein ML: *Wong's Essentials of Pediatric Nursing*, 7th ed. St. Louis: Mosby; 2005:1259.

The use of tools that attempt to quantify the subjective complaint of pain is critical to the ongoing assessment of pain. Figure 14-1 shows several reliable, valid, pain-intensity rating scales with clinical utility. Cognitive impairment may limit the utility of pain-intensity rating scales. The Wong-Baker FACES Pain Rating Scale is useful in MS individuals experiencing both pain and cognitive dysfunction. The pain-intensity rating scales are self-report measures (13,14). Self-report is the gold standard of pain measurement because it is consistent with the definition of pain as a subjective experience (15). The MS nurse must appreciate the fact that self-report measurements are subject to individual differences.

Asking patients to maintain a "pain diary" based on the OLD CART questions is empowering for patients and a useful tool to monitor outcome. Including family members in the assessment is helpful. Parameters of mood, sleep, and quality of life are an objective and ongoing assessment of adequate pain management. The medical outcomes study using Pain Effects Scale (PES) (Table 14-1), part of the Multiple Sclerosis Quality of Life Inventory (MSQLI), is an assessment of the effects of pain on behavior and mood (16).

TABLE 14-1
Pain Effects Scale (PES)

During the past 4 weeks how much did pain interfere with:					
	Not at all	A little	Mode-rately	Quite a bit	To an extreme degree
	1	2	3	4	5
Mood					
Ability to walk or move around					
Sleep					
Normal work (inside and outside the home)					
Recreational activities					
Enjoyment of life					

Add raw scores for a total score (6–30). Higher scores indicate greater impact of pain on ADL and QOL.

The scale reflects the frequency and severity of sensory symptoms on activities of daily living.

Assessment of pain in MS includes (a) self-report measures of pain frequency, quality, and intensity, (b) observational measures from family or significant others of activity level and function, mood, sleep, anxiety, depression, disturbed relationships, or altered role and, (c) physiologic measures such as weight loss, fatigue, depression, or worsening MS.

Mechanism of Multiple Sclerosis Pain

Pain in MS is a direct result of lesions on central nervous system (CNS) myelin, as well as a result of the disability that MS produces relative to disuse of muscles, joints, and tissues (17). Therefore, the pain of MS is mixed, of both neurogenic and nociceptive origin. *Neurogenic pain* is the topic of the following section; *nociceptive pain* arises from a stimulus outside the nervous system. Nociceptive pain is caused by mechanical, thermal, electrical, or chemical insult capable of tissue damage or perceived tissue damage. Nociceptive pain can be acute or chronic. When acute, nociceptive pain serves as a protective mechanism or a wake-up call demanding attention (9,18). A mechanism-based classification that links signs and symptoms of MS pain facilitates mechanism-tailored treatment strategies (19,20).

Neurogenic or Central Pain

Lesions on CNS myelin, which define MS, are the mechanism for the genesis of central neurogenic pain in MS. Neurogenic pain is further described by the character, duration, and intensity of the symptoms experienced. MS neurogenic pain is often experienced independent of any stimulus. Stimulus-independent MS pain is spontaneous and paroxysmal, intermittent or episodic. Such pain is typically characterized as shooting, stabbing, shock-like, lancinating, crushing, or searing. Alternatively, stimulus-independent neurogenic pain can be continuous and described as aching, throbbing, cramping, and burning. Other stimulus-independent abnormal sensations or dysesthesias, are characterized as burning, itching, cold, aching, prickling, tingling, nagging, dull, and band-like. Dysesthesias in MS are typically continuous, with less intensity than those experienced in spontaneous pain syndrome. Yet, ultimately, pain intensity is an individual experience (3,17,19,21).

Neuropathic stimulus-dependent pain is characterized as painful spasms and allodynia. *Allodynia* is pain resulting from a sensation that does not normally cause pain (Table 14-2). Touch, massage, clothing, or the weight of bed covers are painful to persons experiencing allodynia. Stimulus-dependent or evoked pain is usually of short duration and normally lasts only for the period of the stimulus (19,21,22).

Typical neurogenic pain syndromes described in MS includes trigeminal neuralgia, glossopharyngeal neuralgia, episodic facial pain, painful tonic seizures or spasms, dysesthesias of the extremities, thoracic and abdominal band-like sensations, headache, pelvic pain, painful spasticity, episodic facial pain, Lhermitte's phenomenon, and paroxysmal limb pain (3,17,13–25).

Mechanisms of Neurogenic Pain

Lesions on CNS myelin are the responsible mechanisms for neurogenic pain. These lesions cause a disruption in the chemistry and physiology of nerve conduction. Primarily, cell membranes loose their stability. The activation threshold is lowered as sodium channels are created at areas of demyelination, and sodium is upregulated. A lowered threshold accounts for spontaneous and ectopic discharges and ephaptic transmissions or cross-talk, causing axonal sprouting of neurons. Second, there is a loss of inhibitory neurons and neurotransmitters such as endorphins, norepinephrine, and serotonin. Thirdly, an increase occurs in the excitatory neurotransmitters glutamate and aspartate. Excitatory neurotransmitters interact with N-methyl-D-aspartate (NMDA) receptors to allow calcium to enter the cell. Calcium leads to the synthesis of nitric oxide and central sensitization, such that normal sensory input is amplified and sustained. These mechanisms become the rationale for

TABLE 14-2
Pain Definitions

Allodynia. Pain arising from a stimulus that does not normally evoke pain
Analgesia. Absence of pain in response to stimulation that would normally be painful
Dysesthesia. An unpleasant abnormal sensation either spontaneous or evoked
Hyperanesthesia. Increased sensitivity to stimulation
Hyperalgesia. Increased response to a stimulus that is normally painful
Hyperpathia. Painful syndrome of increased reaction to a stimulus and increased threshold
Hypoalgesia. Diminished pain in response to normally painful stimulus
Neuropathic. Disturbance of function or pathologic change in a nerve (peripheral, central, autonomic)
Nociceptor. A receptor sensitive to noxious stimuli
Pain threshold. When a stimulus is perceived as pain
Pain tolerance. Duration or intensity endured before initiating treatment
Paresthesia. An abnormal sensation, whether spontaneous or evolved
Paroxysmal. A recurrent, sudden onset, sharp spasm or convulsion-like

Used with permission from Merskey H, Bogduk N. *International association for the study of pain. Task force on taxonomy. Classification of chronic pain (2nd ed.)* 1994; Seattle, WA: IASP Press, 1994.

TABLE 14-3
Indications for Polypharmacy

Sodium Channel Modulators	NE & 5Ht reuptake inhibitors	Calcium Channel Modulators	NMDA antagonist activity	Increase GABA
Carbamazepine	Imipramine	Gabapentin	Dextromethorphan	Valproate
Oxcarbazepine	Desipramine	Pregabalin	Ketamine	Phenobarbital
Phenytoin	Amitriptyline	Topiramate	Methadone	Baclofen
Mexiletine	Nortriptyline	Zonisamide	Felbamate	Vigabatrin
Lidocaine	Tramadol	Topiramate	Phenobarbital	Tiagabine
Lamotrigine	Duloxetine	Levetiracetam	Topiramate	Benzodiazepines
Zonisamide	Venlafaxine			
Felbamate				
Valproate				

TABLE 14-4
Medications Used to Manage Neurogenic Pain

Agents	Dosage	Adverse Events	Comments
Tricyclic Antidepressants (TCAs)			
Amitriptyline (Elavil)	10 mg daily HS increase by 10 mg weekly to target 150 mg/d	Anticholinergic; sedation, dry mouth, hypotension, blurred vision, weight gain	Act to inhibit reuptake of serotonin and nor-epinephrine; promote sleep, improve mood; use at night; dose-limiting side effects first-line treatment; give at HS, split dosing recommended
Imipramine (Tofranil)	25 mg HS increase by 25 mg weekly to target 300 mg QD	Same as above	
Desipramine (Norpramine)	25 mg HS titrate slowly to target; max 300 mg QD	Better tolerated, fewer anticho-linergic effects	
Nortriptyline (Pamelor)	Same as Elavil		
SNRI Antidepressant Agents			
Duloxetine (Cymbalta)	60 mg 1–2 X/d	Nausea, dizziness, sedation, headache, constipation, dry mouth, fatigue, decreased appetite, increased sweating; liver abnormalities	SSRI/SNRIs may exacerbate flexor spasms (Stolp-Smith et al, 1993) First FDA-approved antidepressant for use in neuropathic pain. Onset 1–4 weeks; use in headache pain; frequent liver function tests required
Venlafaxine (Effexor)	37.5 mg/d, increase by 37.5 mg weekly to target 375 mg QD Extended-release available	GI upset, dizziness, somnolence, insomnia, anorexia, dry mouth, increase sweating, irritability, hypertension	Act to inhibit reuptake of serotonin and norepinephrine; take with food
Antiepileptic Drugs (AEDs)			
Carbamazepine (CBT; Tegretol)	Taper after 3 months use. 100 mg 2X/d with food,	Drowsiness, dizziness, giddiness, dyspepsia,	Raises pain threshold, reduces neuronal hyperexcitability,

(Continued)

TABLE 14-4 (Continued)

	increase slowly to 800–1,000 mg/d Extended release available Bring plasma levels to 6–10 µg/mL	rash, fatigue, double vision, liver toxicity, blood dyscrasias Side effects minimized with long-acting formulas	second-line treatment for neuropathic pain except TN; first-generation, less well tolerated Originally first-line treatment for trigeminal neuralgia; acts to stabilize cell membrane and block sodium channels; plasma level concentration for 50% pain relief is 9.5 µg/mL; need for regular liver function test
Gabapentin (GBT; Neurontin)	300 mg/d increased by 300 mg every 3–5 days to target or maximum 3,600 mg; divided in three daily doses	Headache, dizziness, somnolence, peripheral edema, ataxia, GI upset, incoordination	Second-generation calcium channel blocker; not metabolized, little drug–drug interactions; first-line treatment for neuropathic pain; caution in renal failure; indicated for migraine
Pregabalin (Lyrica)	150 mg 2X/d	Fewer side effects, less fatigue; mild euphoria (schedule V), withdrawal headache and nausea, peripheral edema	Introduced in 2005, FDA-approved for pain; similar to GBT; 2–10 times more potent than gabapentin; no interaction in combination with CBZ, LTG, PHT, VPA
Tiagabine (Gabitril)	4 mg 1X/d, increase weekly by 4 mg to target 56 mg/d in 2 divided doses (MS pain trial maximum dose arbitrarily set at 30 mg/d with mean dose at 12.8 mg/d)	Rash and concentration difficulties	Selective inhibitor of GABA; take with food
Lamotrigine (LMT)	25 mg/d for 2 weeks, titrate slowly	Rash, hypersensitivity reaction,	Blocks sodium channels, inhibits glutamate

(Continued)

TABLE 14-4 (Continued)

(Lamictal)	by 25–50 mg/wk to target 500 mg/d in divided doses	ataxia, double vision, nausea/ vomiting	release; little or no effect on cognitive awareness or arousal; stop drug at first sign of rash; rash may occur at high doses or quick titration; possible seizures; treatment for migraine
Topiramate (Topamax)	50 mg/d increase at 1-week intervals by 50 mg to target 400 mg/d	Drowsiness, cognitive dysfunction, weight loss, fluid retention, kidney stones	Multiple mechanisms of action; greater cognitive dysfunction
Oxcarbazepine (Carbatrol; Trileptal and XR)	Titrate over 4 weeks 600 mg/d to 2.4 g/d in 2 divided doses	Rash, headache, cognitive effects, hyponatremia, nausea/vomiting, double vision, drowsy, dizzy, ataxia	Structurally similar to carbamazepine
Zonisamide (Zonegran)	100 mg/d increased by 100 mg/week to 400 mg/d in divided doses	Drowsiness, anorexia, weight loss, visual hallucinations	Enhances GABA, blocks sodium and calcium channels
Levetiracetam (Keppra)	500 mg 2X/d titrate slowly no higher than 3 g/d	Weight loss, anorexia, cough, spinning sensation	Avoid stopping abruptly; frequent blood studies (hematologic) All anticonvulsants decrease the effectiveness of oral contraceptive agents
Antiarrhythmic Agents			
Mexiletine (Mexitil)	150–600 mg/d in divided doses; maximum 600–900 mg/d	Palpitations, chest pain, tremor, GI upset, dizziness, double vision, nervousness, ataxia, headache	Sodium channel modulator; dose-limiting side effects; good add-on drug

(Continued)

TABLE 14-4 (Continued)

Topical Agents			
Clonidine (Catapres-TTS)	0.1–0.6 mg patches/wk	Dry mouth, drowsiness, dizziness, rash, agitation, constipation, hypotension	Alpha-adrenergic agonist; antagonized by TCAs Rotate sites; local reaction predicts rash with oral dose
Lidocaine (Lidoderm)	5%, 1–3 patches on for 12 hr, off for 12 hr, directly over pain site	Localized irritation, allergic reaction burning, redness, mild tingling	Sodium channel blocker, FDA-approved for pain; use on clean, dry, intact skin
Capsaicin (Zostrix)	A thin film of 0.075% 3X/d-stronger formulas advised to 7.5% for effect		Over-the-counter; apply with gloves; use to reduce oral meds load or oral meds side effects
Fentanyl patch (Duragesic)	12 to 100 μg/hr in 72-hour patch	GI upset, somnolence, apnea, dry mouth, local irritation, headache	Opioid; avoid heat exposure to application site
Nonopioid and Opioid Agents			
Tetrahydro-cannabinol (Dronabinol; Marinol; Sativex in Canada) Tetrahydro-cannabinol/cannabidiol combo and route of dosing produces better effect RCT in progress	10 mg	Dizziness, fatigue, weakness, sleepiness, bad taste, concern for tolerance, addiction	Sativex, an oromucosal (mouth) spray only approved in Canada Not FDA-approved in U.S.; knowledge of long-term safety, potential for dependence, abuse, or misuse unknown
Tramadol (Ultram)	50 mg titrate q wk to a maximum of 100 mg 4X/d or	Sedation, constipation, headache, nausea, dizziness,	Serotonin and norepinephrine reuptake inhibitor; short-acting

(Continued)

TABLE 14-4 (Continued)

	400 mg QD	vertigo	effect; higher doses can produce seizures; habit forming; caution with use of other SSRIs
Morphine sulfate (Kadian, MS Contin, Avinza) Oxycodone (OxyContin, Roxicodone) Hydromorphone, controlled-release (Dilaudid) Hydrocodone (levorphanol; Leco-Dromoran) Meperidine (Demerol) Propoxyphene HCL (Darvon) and combination with nonopioids	Begin with short-acting 5–15 mg every 4 hr and titrate up to efficacy. At 2 weeks, convert to long-acting and use short-acting for breakthrough pain. If doses exceed 180 mg/d see a pain specialist	Sedation, mental clouding, confusion, respiratory depression, nausea and vomiting, constipation, hypotension, confusion, pruritus	For moderate to severe pain; long-acting morphine (Avinza) and (Kadian) fatal in combo with alcohol (use alcohol-free cough syrup) Opioid analgesia; dose dependent Best in conjunction with other neuropathic pain agents; codeine has no known effect in neuropathic pain Meperidine not recommended in chronic pain r/t convulsions
Antispasmodic Agents (Several MS Trials)			
Baclofen (Lioresal)	30 to 120 mg/d, 3 divided doses	Weakness, drowsiness, dizziness, nausea, fatigue, seizures, ataxia, mental confusion	First-line agent for trigeminal neuralgia GABA agonist
Tizanidine (Zanaflex)	2 mg slow titration to 20 mg/d	Sedation, drowsiness, hypotension	Give at HS
Botulinum-A toxin (Botox; Btx-A)	Available in 100-unit vials; 400 units per treatment; 250 U/injection site	Transient site pain on injection and hematoma; muscle weakness	Neurotoxin blocks release of acetylcholine at neuromuscular junction; relief up to 6 months; most useful

(Continued)

TABLE 14-4 (Continued)

	May need repetitive injections		for spasticity of smaller muscles in upper limbs
Selected Nonsteroidal Anti-inflammatory Agents			
Ibuprofen (Motrin; Advil)	400 mg every 4–6 hr; OTC:	GI bleeding, ulcers, stomach pain, fluid retention, hypertension	FDA suggests lowest dose for shortest amount of time; avoid in heart disease, stroke, kidney disease, liver disease
Naproxen (Naprosyn; Aleve)	220 mg every 12 hr Not to exceed 660 in 24 hour; prescription strength: not to exceed 500 mg 2X/d		
Celecoxib (Celebrex)	200 mg 2X/d	Hypersensitivity reaction	Fewer serious GI effects
Aspirin	325–650 mg every 4 hr		
N-Methyl-D-Aspartate (NMDA) Antagonists			
Ketamine (Ketamine/ Midazolam)	PO: 10–25 mg/d to 50 mg/d	Vivid dreams, headache, dizziness, excessive salivation, ataxia, confusion, hallucinations with long-term use, memory impairment, sedation	Receptor antagonists Use in lancinating pain and allodynia Side effects minimize in combination with Midazolam; third-line analgesia
Dextromethorphan and quinidine	5 mg/d titrated to no more than 100 mg/d	Headache, dizziness, spasticity	Off-label combination; currently in Phase II trials for pain and emotional lability
Methadone (Dolophine HCL; Methadose)	Start 5–10 mg 2X/d, increase over 4–7 days by 50% to efficacy; give every 4–6 hr	See Opioids	Inhibits reuptake of serotonin and norepinephrine; binds NMDA receptor; long half-life (190 hr); large volume distribution, unpredictable pharmakinetics; presents dosing challenge; Evidence for use in neuropathic pain; low cost; duration of action 6–12 hr

treating neurogenic pain specific to sodium and calcium channel modulation, NMDA blocking agents, and agents that increase γ-aminobutyric acid (GABA) and the inhibitory neurotransmitters serotonin, norepinephrine, and endorphins (19,20).

Selective Multiple Sclerosis–Related Neurogenic Pain Syndromes

Paroxysmal/Episodic Pain Syndromes

Trigeminal Neuralgia

Trigeminal neuralgia (TN) is a spontaneous, stimulus-independent neurogenic pain experienced by approximately 4% of the MS population, and is 400 times more common in MS than the general population. Trigeminal neuralgia affects one or more branches of the trigeminal nerve that innervates the eye, face, cheek, and jaw. It is an intense, severe, sharp, electric shock–like pain of one side of the eye, face, cheek, or jaw but is more likely to occur bilaterally in people with MS (26). Attacks are spontaneous or can be triggered by a soft breeze, touching, chewing, smiling, tooth-brushing, or any facial movement. Periods of remission follow periods in which sharp, shock-like attacks of between 2 seconds and several minutes occur at varying frequency. In rare instances, the individual experiences a longer duration (45–60 minutes) or, rarely, continuous pain. Trigeminal neuralgia has been known to occur during sleep. In the general population, TN occurs typically after 50 years of age. The presentation of TN in the young adult may indicate underlying demyelinating disease (27).

Trigeminal neuralgia in MS is thought to be associated with a lesion at the trigeminal root entry zone of the pons (28). Interrupting the pain pathway is the mechanism-tailored treatment strategy for TN control in MS. Anticonvulsant medications, known to stabilize cell membranes and decrease the hyperexcitability of sensory neurons via sodium and calcium channel regulation, are first-line treatment for the pain of TN (21,29). The second-generation anticonvulsant agents have milder side-effect profiles. Sustained-released, long-acting formulas minimize side effects. When pain relief is not obtained through drug intervention, surgical gamma knife, radiofrequency, or nerve block procedures that interrupt the pain pathway may become an option. Acupuncture has shown an effect for the pain of TN (30,31).

Headache

Over half (58%) of people with MS suffer episodic headache pain (32). Although the relationship of headache and MS is not entirely clear, MS lesions in the midbrain have been associated with migraine-type headache (33). Headache is seen in people with MS at greater incidence than in the general population, and is usually characterized as a migraine-like, cluster, or tension-type headache. Migraine headache is more commonly reported in patients with relapsing-remitting disease. Some evidence suggests that migraine headaches are associated with exacerbation of MS symptoms (34–35).

Headaches should be treated following existing clinical guidelines for the treatment of headache type. Mechanism-based treatment strategies include increasing the inhibitory neurotransmitters serotonin and norepinephrine. The analgesic properties of tricyclic antidepressants (TCAs)—imipramine, amitriptyline, nortriptyline, and desipramine—have been known for nearly 50 years. Hence, TCAs are the mainstays of treatment for any neurogenic pain, including headache. Tricyclics are the drug class of choice and have a multimodal mechanism of action; basically, they inhibit the reuptake of norepinephrine and serotonin (34). The serotonin and norepinephrine reuptake inhibitors (SNRI) duloxetine and venlafaxine act as neuromodulators of headache pain. Both drugs have proven indications for use in neurogenic pain (36–37). Other SSRIs have not shown efficacy over placebo for neuropathic pain syndromes. Increasing the levels of serotonin and norepinephrine may be an effective ongoing therapy for MS patients experiencing migraine headache, as migraine is linked to changes in serotonin function, and MS patients may have low serotonin levels (35).

Continuous Pain Syndromes in Multiple Sclerosis

Dysesthetic Pain

The most common type of continuous pain experienced in MS is *dysesthetic pain*, defined as an unpleasant, abnormal sensation, either spontaneous or evoked. Dysesthetic pain appears more often in people with minimal MS disability and is characterized as burning, prickling, "pins and needles," tingling, nagging, dull, or band-like sensations (2,17). This persistent pain, often symmetric, affects the legs and feet but may also involve the arms, trunk, and perineum (where it is called vulvodynia). Dysesthetic pain is usually of moderate intensity. Its nagging, persistent nature influences pain tolerance. Dysesthetic pain is worse at night and aggravated by changes in temperature. Dysesthetic pain can be associated with feelings of warmth or cold in the extremities unrelated to actual temperature (17,22). Feeling pain with light touch or the weight of bed sheets and clothing, known as allodynia, is considered the hallmark of stimulus-induced dysesthetic pain. The use of a bed cradle and lambskin pads or booties may offer relief.

Dysesthetic pain is difficult to treat fully. Mechanism-based strategies include neuromodulation and interruption of pain pathways. Tricyclic antidepressants are first-line treatment for dysesthetic pain. Yet, TCAs are often associated with adverse effects (38). Recent evidence suggests that combination therapy (anticonvulsants plus antidepressants) allows for effective pain control by using lower doses of several medications that have different mechanisms of action, thus resulting in fewer side effects (39). Topical agents such as capsaicin (Zostrix), applications of heat and cold, and transdermal agents such as clonidine gel or patch (Catapres-TTS), and the lidocaine patch (Lidoderm) are effective management strategies. Stimulation, in the absence of allodynia, such as fitted prescription pressure stockings at night, massage, acupuncture, acupressure, or transcutaneous electric nerve stimulation (TENS) can offer relief (40).

Nociceptive Pain

Pain in MS unrelated to lesions on CNS myelin occurs as nociceptive pain, specifically pain of muscles, bones, and joints. Nociceptive pain is response to a stimulus that is a mechanical, chemical, thermal or an electrical unpleasant or noxious sensation (9). Nociceptive pain can be intermittent or continuous, provoked or spontaneous. Nociceptive pain involving somatic tissue can be localized and described as aching, squeezing, stabbing, or throbbing. Nociceptive pain involving visceral tissue is not well localized, varies in intensity, and is described as gnawing or cramping, but may be sharp. Visceral pain is often referred to other sites. Nociceptive pain involves real or potential tissue damage and inflammation. Nociceptive pain can be acute or chronic (9,41).

Musculoskeletal

Common nociceptive pain experiences in MS involve the musculoskeletal system and are typically evidenced by back pain and painful spasms. In MS, musculoskeletal pain is a result of weakness, deconditioning, improper use of compensatory muscles, immobility, and stress on bones, muscles, and joints. Steroid use contributes to osteoporosis and possible compromise of the blood supply to large joints (avascular necrosis), with associated pain. Any pain of musculoskeletal nature requires a thorough assessment for lumbar disc disease, avascular necrosis, or other preventive and corrective condition (42).

Prevention is key to the management of musculoskeletal pain. Bone antiresorptive therapies (calcitonin [Miacalcin], risedronate [Actonel], ibandronate [Boniva], alendronate [Fosamax], raloxifene [Evista], teriparatide [Forteo]), smoking cessation, moderate alcohol intake, adequate intake of calcium and vitamin D, fall prevention, and weight-bearing exercise are preventive for pain associated with osteoporosis (43). Physical therapy is an essential primary, secondary, and tertiary intervention for safety, energy conservation, effective movement, positioning, proper seating, and the use of gait aids or joint stabilizers such as ankle-foot orthoses. Exercise and weight control are effective in preventing and treating musculoskeletal pain. Frequent position change and proper support relieve stress on muscles, bones, and joints (42). Acetaminophen (Tylenol), salicylates (aspirin), and nonsteroidal anti-inflammatory agents (NSAIDs) such as ibuprofen (Motrin), naproxen (Aleve), and celecoxib (Celebrex) are first-line oral treatment for musculoskeletal pain. All types of NSAIDs can cause gastrointestinal (GI) irritation and bleeding. NSAIDs decrease renal blood flow and can cause fluid retention and hypertension. NSAID labeling includes a U.S. Food and Drug Administration (FDA) black box warning for the potential for increasing the risk of cardiovascular events and potentially life-threatening GI bleeding. The FDA recommends that NSAIDs be dosed exactly as prescribed or listed on the label. The lowest possible dose should be given for the shortest possible time (44).

Spasticity

Flexor and extensor muscle cramping, pulling, and subsequent pain occurs as spasticity in MS. Spasticity results from a CNS lesion and is exacerbated by noxious stimulation such as a decubitus ulcer, pain, urinary tract infection, or full bowel or bladder. Alleviating the noxious stimuli can minimize spasticity and associated pain. Medical management of pain related to spastic muscles is directed by relieving tonic/clonic muscles with baclofen (Lioresal), tizanidine (Zanaflex), diazepam (Valium), dantrolene (Dantrium), or botulinum toxin (Botox) injection (45).

Pain Management in Multiple Sclerosis

The management of pain in MS involves a combination of medical, behavioral, physical, and surgical interventions (18).

Physical Mechanisms

Physical modalities include physical therapy; stretching; application of heat, cold, and pressure (using prescription pressure stockings); reconditioning to improve strength, endurance and flexibility; counterirritation, such as massage and acupuncture; exercise, such as yoga and t'ai chi; attention to ergonomics and positioning; electroanalgesia, such as TENS; and sound nutrition and weight control.

Behavioral Mechanisms

Cognitive-behavioral approaches to pain management include education, relaxation, behavior modification, distraction, psychotherapy, support groups, imagery, hypnosis, biofeedback, recreation, laugh therapy, music therapy, and, meditation.

Invasive Interventions

Invasive procedures include the intrathecal administration of (either as monotherapy or in combination) baclofen (Lioresal) and morphine, the injection of botulinum toxin (Botox), trigger-point injections, epidural steroids, regional blocks, spinal cord stimulators, and various surgical procedures. *Neuromodulation*, another invasive intervention, uses deep brain stimulation that generates a pulse to relieve pain through electrodes planted in the brain. Neuromodulation has the advantage of being reversible. Evidence suggests that deep brain stimulation is successful for the management of MS neurogenic pain and tremor (46).

Neurosurgical procedures include cordotomy, rhizotomy, percutaneous balloon compression, percutaneous glycerol injection, percutaneous rhizotomy, radiofrequency rhizotomy, and gamma-knife radiosurgery. Microvascular decompression surgery (MVD) has not shown an effect that outweighs side effects for TN pain in MS (47). Neuroablative techniques are considered when medical therapy is not well tolerated or ineffective in managing pain. Quality of life is balanced with possible adverse effects of localized numbness, pain recurrence, and possible worsening of the underlying pain. The presence of sensory loss has been associated with prolonged efficacy in both gamma-knife radiosurgery and glycerol rhizotomy. Percutaneous radiofrequency glycerol rhizotomy is a safe and effective treatment for TN in MS patients, with a reported lower risk of facial sensory loss than other invasive therapies (31,47–49).

Medication Management

Neurogenic Pain

Neurogenic pain is difficult to manage and often resistant to therapy, requiring an in-depth and ongoing assessment of pain indicators, sleep, mood, and quality of life. A mechanistic approach to managing neurogenic pain includes membrane stabilizing agents, NMDA antagonists, dorsal horn inhibitors, increasing GABA activity, and increasing inhibitory neurotransmitters through the use of topical agents, anticonvulsants, antidepressants, antiarrhythmics, NMDA-receptor antagonists, and non-narcotic and narcotic opioids (Figure 14-2).

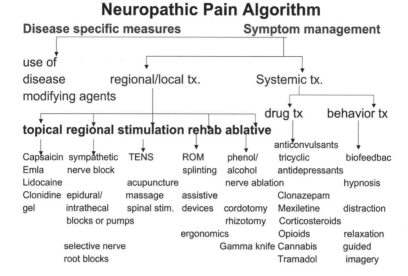

Neuropathic Pain Algorithm

Disease specific measures   **Symptom management**

use of
disease   regional/local tx.   Systemic tx.
modifying agents

drug tx   behavior tx

topical regional stimulation rehab ablative

					anticonvulsants	
Capsaicin	sympathetic	TENS	ROM	phenol/	tricyclic	biofeedbac
Emla	nerve block		splinting	alcohol	antidepressants	
Lidocaine		acupuncture		nerve ablation		hypnosis
Clonidine	epidural/	massage	assistive		Clonazepam	
gel	intrathecal	spinal stim.	devices	cordotomy	Mexiletine	distraction
	blocks or pumps			rhizotomy	Corticosteroids	
			ergonomics		Opioids	relaxation
	selective nerve		Gamma knife	Cannabis	guided
	root blocks			Tramadol	imagery

FIGURE 14-2

Neurogenic pain algorithm.

Nociceptive Pain

Medications used to manage nociceptive pain include salicylates, acetaminophen (Tylenol), NSAIDs, and non-narcotic and narcotic opioids.

Use of Opioids in Neurogenic Pain

The use of opioids for MS neurogenic pain remains controversial, and studies indicate equivocal results (50–51). Rowbotham randomized eight MS patients to either high- or low-dose levorphanol and found a significant effect for the high-dose opioid on pain intensity. The Rowbotham study concluded, however, that the higher, more effective doses produced side effects that had a negative impact on mood and quality of life. The study suggested that reduction in neuropathic pain was similar to that reported in placebo-controlled trials of TCAs and gabapentin (52). In a trial of opioids and gabapentin, gabapentin enhanced the efficacy of morphine analgesic in normal volunteers (53). The advanced practice MS nurse and the MS patient experiencing pain balance the positive and negative aspects of medication therapy and strategize to reach pain control with minimum side effects. The consideration of drug combinations, such as gabapentin and levorphanol, may allow for greater pain control and fewer opioid side effects.

A meta-analysis of several randomized controlled trials demonstrated significant efficacy of opioids over placebo in non-MS neurogenic pain (54).

Studies are needed on the long-term efficacy and safety of opioid use for MS neurogenic pain. Nurses must consider the sedating effect of opioids in MS patients who also experience fatigue. Nurses must also consider the constipating effect of opioids in MS patients who may already struggle with altered bowels function. Initiating a bowel regimen that includes a bowel softener/stimulant combination at bedtime is critical to side-effect management when using opioid analgesia. Opioids have a place in the armamentarium of agents to treat neurogenic pain. Opioids should be considered when other agents become ineffective or not well tolerated (55). Used typically for moderate to severe pain, and used in combination with other adjuvants, opioids can offer neurogenic pain relief. The MS nurse must recognize that, just as pain is a subjective experience, pain management is equally individualized. Individual patients will respond differently to various analgesic therapies. The hallmark of opioid therapy is the need to individualize treatment for each patient: If the prescriber takes into consideration the side effects, the potential for abuse or misuse, and the possibility of drug tolerance, opioid therapy can be a safe and effective treatment for MS neurogenic pain (56).

Use of Cannabis in Neurogenic Pain

Recently, there has been keen interest in the use of marijuana for MS pain management. Cannabis is touted as an effective drug for managing nearly every MS symptom. Studies to date support an effect greater than placebo, but not greater than existing therapies. A large (667 patient) multicenter, randomized, placebo-controlled trial examined the effect of cannabis on spasticity, bladder, tremor, and pain in MS. Trial results were inconclusive, with a perceived improvement in pain (57). Because of the perceived effect on pain, a 5-week study with 66 of the original trial cohort concluded a positive effect of cannabis-based medicine on reducing pain and sleep disorders, with tolerable side effects. Dosing was sublingual and through the oral mucosa (58). The inhaled or smoked form of marijuana is linked to respiratory dysfunction. Evidence also links cannabis with depression, panic attacks, and psychosis. The therapeutic benefit of cannabis may be small compared to its adverse events and unknown toxicity over time, including the potential for abuse and tolerance. The conclusion of MS experts is that there is no evidence to support the use of marijuana for MS symptoms at this time (59). Marijuana is available in oral pill form, dispensed as dronabinol (Marinol) with an indication as an appetite stimulant and antiemetic. It is used off-label as an add-on drug for mild to moderate cancer pain. Anecdotal reports suggest a poor effect of oral cannabinoids on MS pain. An oromucosal form (mouth spray) of cannabis, Sativex, is available in Canada, with indication for pain management effect from multicenter Canadian trials (60). The FDA ruled on medical marijuana in April 2006 saying, "There is sound evidence to support that smoked marijuana is harmful." Marijuana is a schedule 1 substance, the most restrictive schedule of the Controlled Substance Act, meeting criteria for high abuse potential, no currently acceptable medical use, and lack of safety (61). Twelve states have legalized medical marijuana use as of January 2007.

Summary

The goal of pain management is functional, to increase mood, sleep quality, and quality of life. Drug side effects are continually balanced with drug effect. The use of combination therapy or polypharmacy (low doses of different drug classes and different drugs within classes) allows for efficacy while minimizing and increasing the tolerability of drug side effects. Patient education is a key component to medication adherence, allowing patients to maximize function.

Advanced practice MS nurses can assure those patients suffering MS-related pain that pain control is an achievable goal, although the realistic expectation of pain control may be management rather than eradication of pain. Start with a thorough assessment including pain triggers, psychosocial support, and medication history. Use preventive measures and nondrug strategies to supplement, not replace, pharmacologic interventions. Know treatment options and side effects, and treat the side effects. Use low doses of several different medications to achieve better management effect with fewer adverse effects. Begin with low doses and titrate slowly to an effective pain control. If the patient is pain-free for 3 months, titrate back the dosage slowly. It may be possible to discontinue pain medication.

The MS nurse continually surveys patient satisfaction, cognizant of patient outcome measures, mood, sleep, and function or the ability to participate in life.

Pain is a symptom that demands serious attention because it has such a pervasive impact on role, mood, capacity to work and rest, and interpersonal relationships. Untreated pain causes isolation, anger, and depression. Optimum therapeutic treatment involves a commitment to the goal of controlling pain and improving quality of life.

REFERENCES

1. Ehde D, Gibbons L, Chwastiak L, et al. Chronic pain in a large community sample of persons with multiple sclerosis. *Multiple Sclerosis.* 2003;9(6):605–611.

2. Solaro C, Brichetto C, Amato MP, et al. The prevalence of pain in multiple sclerosis. A multicenter cross-sectional study. *Neurology.* 2004;63(5):919–921.

3. Svendsen K, Jensen T, Overvad K, et al. Pain in patients with multiple sclerosis: A population-based study. *Arch Neurol.* 2003;60(8):1089–1094.

4. Ehde D, Osborne T, Jensen M. Chronic pain in persons with multiple sclerosis. Phys Med Rehab Clin N Amer. 2005;16(2):503–512.

5. Kalia l, O'Connor P. Severity of chronic pain and its relationship to quality of life in multiple sclerosis. *Multiple Sclerosis.* 2005;11(3):322–327.

6. Osterberg A, Boivie J, Thuomas KA. Central pain in multiple sclerosis—prevalence and clinical characteristics. *Eur J Pain.* 2005;9(5):531–542.

7. Portenoy RK, Yang K, Thornton D. Chronic intractable pain. An atypical presentation of multiple sclerosis. *J Neurol.* 1988;235:226–228.

8. McCaffery M. Understanding your patient's pain. *Nursing.* 1980;80:26.

9. Merskey H, Bogduk N, and the International Association for the Study of pain, Task Force on Taxonomy. Classification of Chronic Pain, 2nd ed. Seattle: IASP Press, 1994.

10. Ohara PT, Vita JP, Jasmin L. Cortical modulation of pain. *Cell Molecul Life Sci.* 2005;62(1):44–52.

11. Leo J, Huether S. Pain, temperature regulation, sleep, and sensory function. In: K. L. McCance, Huether SE, eds. *Pathophysiology: The Biological Basis for Disease in Adults and Children,* 4th ed. Philadelphia: Mosby; 2005:422–459.

12. Angeles M. In pain, man fires nails into skull. *The Washington Post.* January 28, 2001:A17.

13. Jacox A, Carr D, Payne R, et al. *Managing Cancer Pain: Patient Guide. Clinical Practice Guidelines Number 9 (Adult version-English).* Rockville, MD: U.S. Department of Health and Human Services, Public Health Service, Agency for Healthcare Policy and Research; 1994: AHCPR Publication Number 93–0595.

14. Hockenberry MJ, Wilson D, Winkelstein ML. *Wong's Essentials of Pediatric Nursing,* 7th ed. St. Louis: Mosby, 2004.

15. Strong J, Sturgess J, Unruh A, Vicenzino B. Pain assessment and measurement. In: J Strong, Unruh A, Wright A, Baxter GD, eds. *Pain: A Textbook for Therapists.* Brisbane: Churchill Livingstone, 2001.

16. Ritvo P, Fischer J, Miller D, et al. *Multiple Sclerosis Quality of Life Inventory: A user's manual.* 1997; retrieved on February 1, 2006 from http://www.nationalmssociety.org/pdf/research/MSQLI_Manual_and_Forms.pdf.

17. Moulin D, Foley K, Ebers G. Pain syndromes in multiple sclerosis. *Neurology.* 1988;38:1830–1834.

18. National Pharmaceutical Council (NPC) and Joint Commission on Accreditation of Healthcare Organizations (JCAHO). Pain: Current understanding of assessment, management, and treatments. [Monograph.] 2001; retrieved on January 3, 2006 from http://www.jcaho.org/news+room/health+care+issues/pain_mono_npc.pdf.

19. Hansson PT, Fields HL, Hill RG, Marchettini P, eds. *Progress in Pain Research and Management (Vol. 21). Neuropathic Pain: Pathophysiology and Treatment.* Seattle: IASP Press, 2001.

20. Woolf CJ, Manning RJ. Neuropathic pain: aetiology, symptoms, mechanisms, and management. *Lancet.* 1999;353:1959–1964.

21. Dworkin RH, Backonja M, Rowbotham MC, et al. Advances in neuropathic pain: diagnosis, mechanisms, and treatment recommendations. *Arch Neurol.* 2003;60(11): 1523–1534.

22. Belgrade M. Following the clues to neuropathic pain. Distribution leads reveal the cause and the treatment approach. *Postgrad Med.* 1999;106(6):127–132, 135–140.

23. Stenager E, Knudsen L, Jensen K. Acute and chronic pain syndromes in multiple sclerosis. A five-year follow-up study. *Ital J Neurologic Sci.*, 1995;16:629–632.

24. Miro J, Garcia-Monco C, Leno C, Berciano J. Pelvic pain: An undescribed paroxysmal manifestation of multiple sclerosis. *Pain.* 1988;32:73–75.

25. Minagar A, Sheremata WA. Glossopharyngeal neuralgia in MS. *Neurology.* 2000;54(6): 1368–1370.

26. Hooge J, Redekop W. Trigeminal neuralgia in multiple sclerosis. *Neurology.* 1991;45: 1294–1296.

27. De Simone R, Marano E, Brescia Morra V, et al. A clinical comparison of trigeminal neuralgic pain in patients with and without underlying multiple sclerosis. *Neurologic Sci.* 2005;26 (Suppl. 2):S150–S151.

28. Olafson RA, Rushton JG, Sayre GP. Trigeminal neuralgia in a patient with multiple sclerosis: an autopsy report. *J Neurosurg.* 1966;24(4):755–759.

29. Jensen TS. Anticonvulsants in neuropathic pain: rationale and clinical evidence. *Eur J Pain.* 2002;6(Suppl. A):61–68.

30. Kaufmann A, Patel M. Surgical treatment of trigeminal neuralgia. 2001; retrieved on January 3, 2006 from http://www.umanitoba.ca/centres/cranial.nerves/trigeminal_neuralgia/ manuscript/index.html.

31. Kondziolka D, Lunsford LD. Percutaneous retrogasserian glycerol rhizotomy for trigeminal neuralgia: technique and expectations. *Neurosurg Focus.* 2005;18(5):E7.

32. D'Amico D, La Mantia L, Rigaminti A, et al. Prevalence of primary headache in people with multiple sclerosis. *Cephalalgia.* 2004;24(11):980–984.

33. Gee J, Chang J, Dublin A, Vijayan N. The association of brainstem lesions with migraine-like headache: An imaging study of multiple sclerosis. *Headache.* 2005;45(6):670–677.

34. Rolak L, Brown S. Headaches and multiple sclerosis: A clinical study and review of the literature. *J Neurol.* 1990;237:300–302.

35. Sandyk R, Awerbuch G. The co-occurrence of multiple sclerosis and migraine headache: The serotoninergic link. *Intern J Neurosci.* 1994;76(3–4):249–257.

36. Raskin J, Pritchett YL, Wang F, et al. A double-blind randomized multicenter trial comparing duloxetine with placebo in the management of diabetic neuropathic pain. *Pain Med.* 2005;6(5):346–356.

37. Sumpton JE, Moulin DE. Treatment of neuropathic pain with venlafaxine. *Ann Pharmacotherapeutics.* 2001;35(5):557–559.

38. Sindrup S, Jensen TS. Antidepressants in the treatment of neuropathic pain. In: Hansson PT, Fields HL, Hill RG, Marchettini P, eds. *Neuropathic Pain: Pathophysiology and Treatment (Vol. 21). Progress in pain Research and Management.* Seattle: IASP Press, 2001.

39. Gilron I, Max MG. Combination pharmacotherapy for neuropathic pain: Current evidence and future directions. Expert Rev Neurotherapeutics. 2005;5(6):823–830.

40. Hempenstall K, Nurmikko T, Johnson R, et al. Analgesic therapy for postherpetic neuralgia: A quantitative systematic review. *PLoS Med.* 2005;2(7):e164,0628–0644. Retrieved on January 30, 2006 from www.plosmedicine.org.

41. Moulin D. Pain in central and peripheral demyelinating disorders. *Neurologic Clin.* 1998;16(4):889–898.

42. Maloni H. Pain in multiple sclerosis, an overview of its nature and management. J Neurosci Nurs., 2000;32(3):139–144.

43. Delaney MF. Strategies for the prevention and treatment of osteoporosis during early post-menopause. *Am J Obstet Gynecol.* 2006;194(2 Suppl):S12–S23.

44. Department of Health and Human Services, U.S. Food and Drug Administration, Center for Drug Evaluation and Research. July 18, 2005. COX-2 selective (includes Bextra, Celebrex, and Vioxx) and non-selective non-steroidal anti-inflammatory drugs (NSAIDs). Retrieved on November 29, 2005 from http://www.fda.gov/cder/drug/infopage/cox2/.

45. Beard S, Hunn A, Wight J. Treatments for spasticity and pain in multiple sclerosis: A systemic review. *Health Technol Assess.* 2003;7(40): iii, ix–x, 1–111.

46. Nandi D, Aziz T. Deep brain stimulation in the management of neuropathic pain and multiple sclerosis tremor. *J Clin Neurophysiol.* 2004;21(1):31–39.

47. Eldridge PR, Sinha AK, Javadpour M, et al. Microvascular decompression for trigeminal neuralgia in patients with multiple sclerosis. *Stereotactic Functional Neurosurg.* 2003;81 (1–4):57–64.

48. Pickett G, Bisnaire D, Ferguson G. Percutaneous retrogasserian glycerol rhizotomy in the treatment of tic douloureux associated with multiple sclerosis. *Neurosurgery.* 2005;56(3): 537–545.

49. McNatt SA, Yu C, Giannotta SL, et al. Gamma knife radiosurgery for trigeminal neuralgia. *Neurosurg.* 2005;56(6):1295–1301.

50. Kalman S, Osterberg A., Sorenson J, et al. Morphine responsiveness in a group of well-defined multiple sclerosis patients: A study with i.v. morphine. *Eur J Pain.* 2002;6(1):69–80.

51. Rowbotham MC. Efficacy of opioids in neuropathic pain. In: Hansson PT, Fields HL, Hill RG, Marchettini P, eds. *Neuropathic Pain: Pathophysiology and Treatment (Vol. 21). Progress in Pain Research and Management.* Seattle: IASP Press, 2003.

52. Eckhardt K, Ammon S, Hofmann U, et al. Gabapentin enhances the analgesic effect of morphine in healthy volunteers. *Anesthesia Analgesia.* 2000;91(1):85–191.

53. Rowbotham MC, Twilling L, Davies PS, et al. Oral opioid therapy for chronic peripheral and central neuropathic pain. *N Engl J Med.* 2003;348:1223–1232.

54. Eisenberg E, McNicol E, Carr D. Efficacy and safety of opioid agonists in the treatment of neuropathic pain of nonmalignant origin. Systemic review and meta-analysis of randomized controlled trials. *JAMA.* 2005;293:3042–3052.

55. Guarino A, Cornell M. Opioids as a treatment option for MS patients with chronic pain. *Intern J MS Care.* 2005:Spring:10–15.

56. Coluzzi F, Pappagallo M. Opioid therapy in chronic noncancer pain: Practice guidelines for initiation and maintenance of therapy. *Minerva Anestesioligica.* 2005;71:425–433.

57. Zajicek J, Fox P, Sander H, et al., and the UK MS Research Group. Cannabinoids for the treatment of spasticity and other symptoms related to multiple sclerosis (CAMS study): Multicenter, randomized, placebo controlled trial. *Lancet.* 2003;362:1517–1526.

58. Rog D, Nurmikko T, Friede T, Young C. Randomized controlled trial of cannabis-based medicine in central pain in multiple sclerosis. *Neurology.* 2005;65(6):812–819.

59. Unpublished, Cannabis Task Force. New York: National Capital Multiple Sclerosis Society, October 16, 2006.

60. Perrac C. Sativex for the management of multiple sclerosis symptoms. *Issues Emerging Health Technol.* 2005;72:1–4.

61. U.S. Food and Drug Administration inter-agency advisory regarding claims that smoked marijuana is a medicine. April 2006; retrieved on January 20, 2007 from http://www.fda.gov/bbs/topics/NEWS/2006/NEW01362.html.

CHAPTER 15

Depression in MS Assessment and Treatment

June Halper

Over the past decade, the community of multiple sclerosis (MS) healthcare professionals has recognized that the incidence and prevalence of depression in MS exceeds previous estimates (1). Although initially thought to be a reaction to the diagnosis of a disabling condition, subsequent work has shown depression is significantly more common with MS than those similarly disabled by other chronic diseases. Estimates have ranged from 14% to 57%, and the lifetime prevalence in an individual with MS is reported to be as high as 50% (2,3). Several studies have shown that the risk of suicide is significantly higher for a patient with MS than in a matched control (4). There has been speculation that genetic factors, a structural cause, or a relationship to the inflammatory process may be present (1).

The review of the literature reveals that, while treatment of depression is a critical component in the management of MS, almost no information is available about patterns of treatment. Estimates about depression conclude that more than half of depressed patients do not receive the recommended dose or duration for pharmacotherapy. The findings of Schiff and colleagues are of great interest, and seem to suggest that depression may be part of the disease (5). Despite the high prevalence of mood illness in MS as compared to those with no psychiatric disorder, first-degree relatives do not have a high prevalence of mood disorders. Therefore, mood disorder in MS does not appear to conform to familial patterns of primary mood disorder (6). Evidence appears to indicate a strong association with bipolar disorder as well. This association does not appear to be a reaction to MS disability nor does it seem to follow a familial pattern in the primary disorder (7). Although there has been a great deal of interest in the relationship of interferon therapy and depression, there has been no conclusive evidence to support this conclusion (8).

It is imperative, as with any symptom of MS, that this problem is assessed and treated appropriately and dynamically. Depressive symptoms, sadness, tearfulness, irritability, hopelessness, and withdrawal are experienced by everyone at some time in their lives. A patient may lose not only the normal capacity to function, but also roles in family, society, usual work, leisure activity, and relationships. Depression related to MS involves a sustained period of depressed mood, loss of interest in life, changes in appetite, sleep disturbance, and psychomotor retardation. There may be feeling of worthlessness and thoughts of suicide. Suicidal ideation or a plan to end one's life must be treated immediately and on an ongoing basis. Vigilant monitoring is essential for signals that indicate that the patient is suffering from extreme depression and hopelessness.

Assessing depression in an MS population is a challenge because most instruments have been developed for a mental health population. These have included Beck's Depression inventory, the Schedule for Affective Disorders, and the Self-Rating Depression Scale. None of these scales has been documented as appropriate for MS, and no clinical practice guidelines have been generated for clinical use. The Goldman Consensus Group published the results of their study of this problem (9) and have generated an algorithm that still remains a work in progress. The conclusion thus far is that assessment of depression should be an integral part of MS management throughout the lifetime with the disease. The most effective management of depression is a combination of pharmacologic intervention and psychosocial supports.

Implications for Care

As we know, MS affects the entire family. Family members may be called upon to provide emotional and practical support; they also have to deal with disappointment, uncertainty, role reversals, and financial burdens due to the illness itself and potentially reduced income. The nurse, when assessing for depression, should inquire about family coping and for signs of depression in family members. Children are particularly vulnerable and may become anxious and fearful of the future (10).

As with all other symptoms of MS, a comprehensive approach appears to work most effectively. A combination of psychotherapy and antidepressant medications has been shown to be more efficacious than either intervention alone (11). Structured psychotherapy with either a social worker or psychologist is usually effective; with significant psychiatric difficulties, a psychiatric referral may be more appropriate.

Regardless of the provider, issues related to MS include:

- Dealing with the new diagnosis and the psychological pain of an exacerbation
- Addressing loss of function and diminished self-esteem
- Acknowledging and dealing with role changes and conflicts about loss of independence
- Apprehension about the future

These issues can be addressed as they occur, if they do, by knowledgeable healthcare professionals who are concerned and appreciate the extent of loss one may experience. Some people prefer and benefit from group therapy. There is some evidence that therapeutic groups may improve patients' abilities to cope with the illness and may reduce depression (12).

Couples and family members often find it useful to talk with a mental health professional or their medical team. If family dysfunction is severe, family therapy is indicated. Therapists may help them understand the root of their problems, problem-solve to develop effective strategies, and minimize blame and guilt that may arise due to MS.

Pharmacotherapy

Antidepressants have been used successfully in the management of depression. The tricyclic medications such as amitriptyline and imipramine were used successfully in the latter part of the 20th century. The addition of selective serotonin reuptake inhibitor (SSRI) and selective norepinephrine reuptake inhibitors (SNRI) anti-depressants improved successful management of this symptom (Table 15-1). The Goldman Consensus Group emphasized the potential effectiveness of increasing dosages and the potential benefit of combination therapy (9).

Summary

Depression in MS is extremely common throughout a lifetime with the disease. It may be circumstantial, related to the uncertainty of the disease itself, or it may be a symptom of the dynamic changes caused by MS. In either event, healthcare professionals are challenged to assess and treat this problem throughout the course of the illness and to be vigilant for its presence.

TABLE 15-1
Common Antidepressant Medications Used in MS

Brand Name	Generic Name	Additional Comments
Common Tricyclic Antidepressants		
Elavil	Amitryptiline	May also be used for neuropathic pain
Norpramin	Desipramine	Approved for OCD
Sinequan	Doxepin	
Tofranil	Imipramine	Depression, bladder dysfunction
Pamelor	Nortriptyline	
Selective Serotonin Reuptake Inhibitors (SSRI)		
Celexa	Citalopram	
Lexapro	Escitalopram	
Paxil	Paroxetine	Regular and extended release available
Prozac, Prozac weekly, Sarafem	Fluoxetine	May be effective in fatigue
Zoloft	Sertraline	
Serotonin/Norepinephrine Reuptake Inhibitors (SNRI)		
Cymbalta	Duloxetine	Approved for diabetic related neuropathic pain
Effexor	Venlafaxine	
Dopamine Reuptake Blocking Agents		
Wellbutrin, Wellbutrin SR, Wellbutrin XL, Zyban	Bupropion	Contraindicated in seizures

REFERENCES

1. McGuigan C, Hutchinson M. Unrecognised symptoms of depression in a community-based population with multiple sclerosis. *J Neurology*. 2006;253:219–223.
2. Patten SB, Metz LM, Reimer MA. Biopsychosocial correlates of lifetime major depression in a MS population. *Multiple Sclerosis*. 2000;6:115–120.
3. Sadovnick AD, Remick RA, Allen J, et al. Depression and multiple sclerosis. *Neurology*. 1996;46:628–632.
4. Sadovnick AD, Eisen K, Paty DW, Ebers GC. Cause of death in patients attending multiple sclerosis clinica. *Neurology*. 1991;41:1193–1196.
5. Mohr DC, Hart SL, Fonareva I, Tasch ES. Treatment of depression for patients with multiple sclerosis in neurology clinics. *Multiple Sclerosis*. 2006;12:204–208.

6. Gershon JED, Bunney WE, Leckman JF. The inheritance of affective disorders: A review of data hypotheses. *Behav Genet.* 1976;6:227–261.

7. Joffe RT, Lippert GP, Gray TA, et al. Mood disorder in multiple sclerosis. In: Jensen K, Knudsen Stenager JE, Grant I, eds. *Mental Disorders and Cognitive Deficits in Multiple Sclerosis.* London: John Libbey, 1989.

8. Galeazzi GM, Ferrari S, Giaroli G, et al. Psychiatric disorders and depression in multiple sclerosis outpatients: Impact of disability and interferon beta therapy. *Neurol Sci.* 2005;26:4,255–262.

9. Goldman Consensus Group. The Goldman Consensus statement on depression in multiple sclerosis. *Multiple Sclerosis.* 2005;11:328–337.

10. Minden SL, Moes E. A psychiatric perspective. In: Rao SM, ed. *Neurobehavioral Aspects of Multiple Sclerosis.* New York: Oxford University Press; 1990: 230–250.

11. Weissman MM. The psychological treatment of depression. Evidence for the efficacy of psychotherapy alone, in comparison with, and in combination with pharmacotherapy. *Arch Gen Psychiat.* 1979;36:1261–1269.

12. Crawford JD, McIvor GP. Group psychotherapy: Benefits in multiple sclerosis. *Arch Phys Med Rehabil.* 1985;66:810–813.

CHAPTER 16

Skin Care in Multiple Sclerosis

June Halper

Historically, nurses specializing in multiple sclerosis (MS) care have focused on skin care in terms of prevention of skin breakdown due to prolonged immobility, poor body alignment, and even inadequate nutrition. Nursing education has been more than adequate in preparing us for these complications and, although these still occur in multiple sclerosis, new rehabilitation techniques, products, technology, and pharmacologic innovations have provided us with an expanded armamentarium of tools and skills.

Disease-modifying therapies (DMTs) have altered the landscape of MS care and added to the need for skills development in patients and their families. Frequent self-injections pose substantial challenges to physicians, nurses, and the roster of those who are initiating and sustaining therapy. Adherence literature clearly points to indicators of successful medication regimes that pro vide patients with an acceptable level of comfort and a minimal level of anxiety due to complications. Since the early 1990s, with the advent of these therapies, the focus has been on adverse events with injectables (quality of life, flu-like symptoms, fatigue). Although these can be debilitating, it is essential that we acknowledge that the more visible symptoms of skin reaction not be neglected. A person's self image and acceptance of a chronic illness or disability can be disrupted by highly visible evidence of underlying problems.

Once a person is started on an injectable therapy, there is the danger that clinicians will take for granted that the proper technique is being used and that there are no complications that impede adherence. It is imperative that nothing should be taken for granted; ongoing vigilance will ensure that the benefits of therapy will be sustained. In addition to issues of skin care, it is important to acknowledge that many people have self-injection anxiety. This should be assessed and addressed right from the outset. Many strategies for this problem have been identified in the literature and strategies have been developed to cope with it. One recent study described the development of a program that allayed fears, reframed the patient's perceptions of injectable therapies (cognitive reframing), dealt with the vasovagal response and an aversion to injectables, and managed pain and side effects (1).

As an obvious impediment to adherence to injectable therapy, skin reactions to DMTs can take a variety of forms and can range in severity from mild irritation to severe infections. It is the role of the clinician to educate the patient on appropriate skin care and to routinely inspect a patient's skin to look for any sign that a "refresher" course is needed on their injectable therapy. All approved therapies have immunogenic properties, so it is not surprising that skin reactions are common occurrences, whether a mild burning sensation or a full-blown skin reaction. It is important to acknowledge that most injection reactions occur with subcutaneous (SC) injections rather than with intramuscular (IM) delivery. These reactions include erythema and edema along with pruritus that may be self-limited or persistent.

In addition to these mild reactions, a small number of patients experience the cosmetic problem of lipoatrophy, characterized by irregular areas of skin depression, similar in appearance to cellulite. Lipoatrophy is believed to be caused by damage to fat cells from frequent injections. It can be very disfiguring, and is believed to be permanent. This can have a significant psychological impact on body image (2).

Certain factors influence the occurrence of skin reactions. These may be patient-related in terms of injection technique, or physiologically related in terms of skin color, texture, weight, and gender (darker skinned people have decreased occurrence of skin reactions but tend to scar; hairier body areas that are injected can develop more infections; thinner people tend to have more difficulty with lipoatrophy; women tend to have more lipoatrophy than men). It is very important to screen patients for pre-existing dermatologic problems (eczema, psoriasis, hypersensitive skin problems) when initiating injectable therapy.

Injection site selection can also influence the development of skin reactions. Injecting into the same site repeatedly, without site rotation, can lead to problems. Some patients routinely inject in an area that is convenient or that has sensory loss secondary to MS; this can result in permanent skin damage to that particular site.

Patients and clinicians can take a number of measures to minimize skin reactions. The most crucial is ongoing reinforcement of injection technique. It is not adequate to educate patients and care partners when therapy is begun: Repeated reiteration of the importance of site rotation and awareness of possible reactions is equally important to prevent long-term complications and skin reactions.

Needle selection is important in injectable therapy. A key principle is to try to use the appropriate needle size and length for the prescribed injectable. For example, it is obvious that longer needles are appropriate for IM injection whereas, on the whole, shorter needles are appropriate for SC injection. However, there are some exceptions. For patients with thin arms and less muscle mass, a shorter needle might be suitable for an IM injection. On the other hand, patients with excess subcutaneous fat may benefit from a longer needle for SC administration (3). Similarly, needle length should be adjusted for areas of the body that have more or less tissue. Although some people inject manually, the use of the auto-injector with SC injections makes this process easier, because the depth of needle penetration can be reset for different sites. Patients may have to be instructed on various needle depths when learning how to do injections.

Pain and burning are common reactions to injectable medications, and these can be ameliorated by warming the medication to room (or perhaps body) temperature. Brief application of ice to the injection site (30 seconds) can reduce painful injections. Applying a topical anesthetic, such as the lidocaine-based agents EML Aor LMX, for approximately 30 minutes prior to injection can reduce pain and burning (4). However, it is essential that the cream be washed off before injecting to avoid introducing the cream into the injection site. Similarly, alcohol should be allowed to dry before injecting. Perfumed moisturizers should be avoided on potential injection sites. Soap and water cleansing is used in Europe and is quite adequate for skin preparation, but it important to keep in mind that the area must be thoroughly dry before injecting (4). A recent study investigating the use of warm compresses with administration of Copaxone found clinical benefit (5).

Frequently, patients believe that they have to expel air bubbles from the syringe prior to the injection. This involves pushing some of the diluent out of the tip of the needle. This should be avoided, because the solution at the tip of the needle can be irritating to the skin. Injections sites should remain covered when out in the sunlight because exposure to the sun can result in hardening and drying of the skin, making injections more difficult at that site. It has also been postulated that smokers may be susceptible to increased skin reactions because chronic use of nicotine can result in peripheral vasoconstriction (4).

Regular site rotation is one of the most critical elements in minimizing skins problems. It is recommended that sites be rotated by using one limb (arm or leg) for an injection and then subsequently inject in the opposite leg or arm. Sites such as the buttocks can be accessed by a care partner, thus increasing areas of injection. Repeated injection in the same site can lead to long-term problems. It is not enough to inject 1 inch away from a previous site it is critical to avoid using the same site within the same week. This may involve enlisting the help of a care partner to assist in using less accessible sites such as the buttocks and sides of the hips.

Injection site reactions are expected in SC delivery of medication. Frequently, patients complain of red raised areas that become pruritic and remain so for an extended period. If redness and raised injection sites occur immediately after injection, this is an immediate histamine reaction and can be managed with oral antihistamine therapy (either over-the-counter Benadryl or prescription Zyrtec). If this reaction is delayed, a topical mid-potency steroid cream can manage the problem. Mid-potency steroids are available by prescription (4).

The patient's skin should be inspected at each visit with an assessment (verbal is adequate) of how they are injecting. At times, it might be necessary for the patient to demonstrate his technique, particularly when skin reactions are becoming a more frequent problem.

As with all aspects of managing MS, nurses must keep the lines of communication open. Some patients are reluctant to acknowledge problems because they may be concerned that their medication will be discontinued. Other patients may just accept skin reactions because they believe they are unavoidable results of self-injecting.

Summary

Tips for managing skin reactions with frequent injectable therapies in MS:

- Be aware of potential skin problems including erythema, pain, burning, edema, and the potential for lipoatrophy.
- Educate and reeducate patients on proper injection technique.
- Assess patients for potential pre-existing conditions that may be exacerbated by the properties of DMTs in MS.
- Ensure that the medication is at room temperature prior to injection.
- Avoid introducing alcohol, perfumed soaps, moisturizers into the injection site.
- Emphasize the importance of site rotation.
- Numb injection site to reduce pain (ice, topical anesthetics).
- Wipe injection site dry before injecting.
- Adjust needle lengths appropriately.
- Routinely inspect injection sites.
- Observe self-injection technique when problems occur.

REFERENCES

1. Cox D, Stone J. Managing self-injection difficulties in patients with multiple sclerosis. *J Neurosci Nurs.* 2006;38(3):167–171.
2. Habif TJ. *Clinical Dermatology.* New York: Mosby, 2003.

3. Jolley H, et al. The use of warm compresses with Copaxone injection. Poster presentation. CMSC Annual Meeting. Phoenix, AZ. June 2006.

4. Machler B. Skin care in MS. Personal communication, 2006.

5. Buhse M. Efficacy of EMLA cream to reduce fear and pain association with interferon beta-1a injection in multiple sclerosis. *J Neurosci Nurs.* 2006;38(4):222–226.

CHAPTER 17

Complementary and Alternative Therapies

Patricia M. Kennedy

The use of unconventional therapies is common among the general population, but it is believed to be higher among people living with multiple sclerosis (MS). As nurses, we often serve as an information resource for our patients, so it is imperative that we become knowledgeable and comfortable with the concept of complementary and alternative medicine (CAM).

Definitions

+ Unconventional therapies are usually described as therapies not generally taught in medical schools or available in hospitals.
+ Conventional therapies are those that are taught in medical schools and are available in hospitals. These would all fall under the headings of medicine, surgery, rehabilitation, psychology, and dietetics.
+ Complementary medicine is the use of conventional medicine with unconventional medicine.
+ Alternative medicine is unconventional medicine used instead of conventional therapy.

TABLE 17-1
Why Patients with Multiple Sclerosis Use Complementary
and Alternative Medicine

✦ Conventional medicine does not have all the answers
✦ Available conventional therapies may be limited in number or too costly
✦ Patients want to do all they can to promote their own health
✦ MS is chronic, usually progressive and no cure is yet available
✦ Some patients mistrust the medical establishment
✦ Some patients make decisions based on emotions, hearsay, and poor or erroneous information

CAM therapies change over time. Because traditional medical practitioners are utilizing CAM therapies in their treatment of illnesses and conditions, these methods are becoming more conventional. Pregnant women are advised to take prenatal vitamins and folic acid supplements; patients who have had a myocardial infarction are advised to exercise, follow specific nutritional guidelines, and learn stress management techniques. Acupuncture might be recommended as a part of a total program of pain management.

Use of Complementary and Alternative Medicine

In international studies, the use of CAM in people with MS has been found to be as high as 50% to 60%. Multiple sclerosis patients are found to usually use unconventional therapy in conjunction with conventional therapy (Table 17-1). The more commonly used therapies are special diets, supplements, prayer and spirituality, chiropractic medicine, and massage.

Appropriate Use of Complementary and Alternative Medicine

In the treatment of MS, conventional therapies are available that have gone through rigorous clinical trials, and their benefit for disease modification has been measured scientifically and without bias. These disease-modifying agents are interferon beta-1b, interferon beta-1a (IM), interferon beta-1a (SC), and glatiramer acetate. Also included in this class is mitoxantrone. In spite of the fact that none of these treatments is 100% effective and that they often cause significant side effects, patients should never be advised to utilize an alternative therapy that has no similar scientific evidence to support its effectiveness instead of conventional treatment. However, patients may choose an alternative therapy to augment their treatment.

By the same token, severe symptoms seen in MS should be treated with therapies known, through scientific investigation, to be effective and safe. Such symptoms include severe spasticity, depression, urinary tract infections (UTIs), pressure ulcers, and pain. Existing conventional treatments are not always 100% effective, however, and the use of unconventional therapies may be utilized in conjunction with conventional therapy. Mild symptoms may be managed with a CAM therapy alone.

Evidence-Based Approach to Medical Care

Evidence-based medicine (EBM) has been defined by David Sackett as "the conscientious, explicit, and judicious use of current best evidence in making decisions about the care of individual patients. The practice of evidence based medicine means integrating individual clinical expertise with the best available external clinical evidence from systematic research" (1). More recently, he described it as the "integration of best research evidence with clinical expertise and patient values" (2).

Evidence Available for Conventional Therapies for Multiple Sclerosis

Medications available by prescription have been rigorously studied and are not available to patients until the U.S. Food and Drug Administration (FDA) (or similar regulatory body in countries outside the United States) has granted approval. Some conventional therapies for MS symptoms and disease modification may be only partially effective and may be limited by side effects. Other therapies used to treat disease or symptoms are recommended without evidence for use in MS (off-label use) (3).

Evidence Available for Complementary and Alternative Medicine

Clinical studies of unconventional therapies are seldom done, and when undertaken, they utilize small numbers of participants compared to the large, multicenter clinical trials performed for conventional medications. Part of the reason is that some therapies have little obvious *scientific* rationale (such as reflexology), thus making it difficult to evaluate them objectively. Some treatments, such as massage or yoga, are difficult to study with control subjects using a placebo. Alternative treatments are generally not patentable, so there is no financial incentive for doing an expensive, well-designed clinical study.

TABLE 17-2
How Medical Professionals Respond to the Use of CAM in Their Patients

✦ **Don't ask:** They don't believe in CAM, don't want to know, or consider it not important enough to take up time. Lines of communication are closed.
✦ **Don't discuss:** They don't believe in CAM, so spending time on it is not appropriate, or they may have limited information about CAM use and are unable to discuss. Communication about CAM in the future will not be forthcoming from the patient.
✦ **Dismiss:** They disagree with CAM use and let patient know their beliefs and ideas are not as valuable as the provider's. They may not be knowledgeable. Patient feels discounted and will not discuss with the provider again.
✦ **Discuss:** They hear what the patient is practicing or considering. They offer information, if known, or look it up if not known. Communication linews are open, benefiting both provider and patient.
✦ **Recommend:** They actually make recommendations about specific treatments or practitioners for use by patients. Providers must be well informed about risks and benefits before recommending any therapy, including CAM. Recommendations for CAM practitioners must be made with the same scrutiny that would be used for referral to any healthcare provider.

Placebo Effect

Many medical professionals view some CAM as placebo treatment and, by so doing, eliminate any credibility applicable to that treatment (Table 17-2). Since the advent of randomized, placebo-controlled clinical trials, *placebo* has taken on new meaning. Placebos used to be given to patients as treatment by their physicians. Because patients trusted their physicians, the treatments given by them had strong benefit because of the therapeutic liaison existing between patient and doctor. It became unethical to prescribe placebos when proven therapies are available. The practice of medicine, then, became more science than art. Providers now spend less time with patients, and patients are less likely to adhere to physician recommendations. Patients may look elsewhere for treatment for their illnesses (what the patient feels and suffers), while healthcare providers become more focused on the disease (what the doctor sees and finds).

Placebo response is the behavioral change in the person receiving the treatment and *the placebo effect* is that part of the change attributable to the symbolic effect of the treatment (4). Placebo response has also been defined as "a change in the body that occurs as the result of the symbolic significance that oneattributes to an event or object in the healing environment" (4). The

TABLE 17-3

How to Work with Patients Who Utilize CAM

✦ Ask routinely what medications, herbs, vitamins, supplements, and other treatments they use
✦ With CAM use, incorporate it into the treatment plan if appropriate. If not appropriate, explain the reasons to the patient.
✦ Assess the response to CAM that a patient might exhibit or describe just as you would any therapy. Provide feedback to the patient, both positive and negative, and document it in the record.
✦ Continue to provide accurate information when able, but explain when there is no information available to you.

placebo effect highlights the difference between the art and science of medicine. Doctors look for a cure, but patients still want care (4). Placebos can actually effect physiologic changes seen in many clinical trials using a placebo arm.

Patients seek care wherever they can get it; some believe that, because some CAM practitioners spend more time with the patient, the patient gains more benefit from the treatment he receives. Convincing anecdotal stories about how others have felt better using a particular treatment sways other patients. If a patient experiences physical or psychological improvement from their choice of CAM therapies, it is important for professional care providers to not to diminish or ridicule this effect. Counsel patients about any harmful effects or interactions, if known, but otherwise, incorporate their choices in the treatment plan (Table 17-3).

Are Alternative Therapies Safe?

Each therapy must be evaluated individually. In general though, teach patients that "natural" does not always mean "good for you." Some supplements, such as comfrey and chaparral, are known to be unsafe and should be avoided.Likewise, over-the-counter (OTC) does not always mean safe. Acetaminophen can be toxic if taken in amounts exceeding the recommended doses. In addition, the safety of OTC therapies can depend on several things:

+ What is in the product?
+ Where do the ingredients come from?
+ What is the quality of the manufacturing?

+ Are the ingredients known? If the ingredients are said to be proprietary, the contents are not usually made known.

The response to any therapy, conventional or unconventional, varies among individuals. Encourage patients to report side effects or adverse reactions to any therapy.

If the CAM product is a dietary supplement (a product taken by mouth that contains a "dietary ingredient" intended to supplement the diet), or a natural health product (in Canada), the manufacturer of that product is solely responsible for the safety and effectiveness of the product. In the United States, the FDA has no authority over the quality of the dietary supplements. The FDA can, however, remove a product from the marketplace if the product has been reported to the FDA as potentially harmful, and their research has determined it to be dangerous to the health. The FDA also defines the labeling or marketing of a supplement. Any product that claims an ability to diagnose, treat, cure, or prevent disease is considered a drug, and selling it is illegal unless it goes through the same evaluation as any other drug. In 1999, the Canadian Office of Natural Health Products (ONHP) was established. It requires a premarketing approval process for the safety of products and requires reasonable evidence for product claims. It has developed guidelines for surveillance of adverse events, and it does post-approval monitoring of alternative therapies. ONHP licenses and inspects manufacturing facilities and determines what information should be included on product labels. It is also charged with providing information for Canadian consumers to assist them in decisions about CAM.

Further sources of information on CAM is listed in Table 17-4.

Assisting Patients in Choosing Complementary and Alternative Medicine

When discussing the use of CAM therapy with your patients, ask them the following questions:

+ Is there any evidence (scientific, not anecdotal) that the treatment is helpful?
+ Is there any evidence that the treatment is harmful?
+ Does it sound too good to be true?
+ Is it affordable by the patient and accessible to the patient?
+ Are there claims that the therapy cures or treats a wide range of unrelated diseases?

They can always use these questions themselves when making decisions in the future.

TABLE 17-4
Sources of Information for Patients Wanting to Use CAM

Books: Many books are available to patients in libraries, in stores that sell CAM products, and in bookstores. Unfortunately, the information available in them is inconsistent and at times incorrect. As nurses, having a list of reliable resources for your patients is helpful.
Commercials and infomercials: Marketing can be persuasive. Teach patients how to tell the difference between anecdotal information and information with scientific merit.
Peers and support groups: Whenever two or more are gathered, it seems that everyone likes to exchange ideas on managing illness. Although well-meaning, the information is not always based on safety or fact. Talk with your patients about how to manage that type of information.
Online: Although many extremely informative and factual web sites exist, there are equally as many web sites with biased or erroneous information. Offer your patients a handout with reliable web sites.
Alternative practitioners: Many practitioners are willing to work with healthcare providers in planning a truly complementary care plan for patients. Patients feel very supported when this occurs. It would be wise to counsel patients about any provider, either medical or alternative, who make claims that "his way is the only way".
Medical professional: Healthcare providers should be comfortable when patients come to them seeking information and advice. Discussion should include a review of side effects, interactions with medications (prescribed and over the counter), risks, and known benefits. If the healthcare provider is not open to the discussion, the patient is not likely to ever discuss it with them again. Nurses should be open to these questions and do all they can to provide the answers.

Classifications of Complementary and Alternative Medicine

Complementary and alternative medicine (CAM) therapies are classified according to the National Institutes of Health's National Center for Complementary and Alternative Medicine:

+ Alternative medical systems. These include complete systems of theory and practice. Such systems include traditional Chinese medicine, Ayurveda, homeopathic medicine, and naturopathic medicine.
+ Mind-body interventions. These techniques were designed to enhance the mind's ability to affect the body and its functions. These techniques include prayer, meditation, mental healing, and an array of other methods such as music, dance, and art.

+ Biologically based therapies. These include substances found in nature, such as herbs, foods, and vitamins. Dietary supplements, herbal products, diets, and vitamin therapy fall into this category.
+ Manipulative and body-based methods. These techniques include manipulation and/or movement of one or more parts of the body. Chiropractic, osteopathy, and massage are included in these techniques. Also included are yoga and t'ai chi.
+ Energy therapies. These therapies involve the use of energy fields. One type, biofield therapies, has effect on energy fields that surround and penetrate the body. Scientifically, the presence of these fields has not been proven. Examples of these therapies include therapeutic touch, Reiki, and qi gong. Another type of energy therapy is bioelectromagnetics-based. These involve using electromagnetic fields to effect benefit on disease or symptoms.

Sometimes included in CAM classification are those methods used for lifestyle changes and disease prevention. Whether they are considered in the realm of unconventional therapy or in the realm of conventional medical practice, they are widely used. Healthcare providers must be aware of patient practices, and may make recommendations for some of these methods. Some of these methods include exercise, stress management, nutrition, sleep hygiene, and weight management.

Helping Your Patients with Web Site Information

The Internet is a wonderful way for patients and healthcare professionals alike to stay abreast of new treatment methods. Because of the wealth of information found on the Internet, it has become a commonly used resource for making healthcare decisions. When your patients use the Internet for information about CAM products, methods, or therapies, offer them a few guidelines. NCCAM recommends the following questions:

+ Whose site is it? Academic institutions, professional associations, government agencies, or well-respected MS organizations are likely to provide balanced and factual material. If the web site is owned by a commercial endeavor, information about their product may be biased toward selling it.
+ Why does the site exist? Education or marketing?
+ What is the basis of the information? Scientific evidence with clear references, or testimonials and opinion?
+ How current is the information? Is it reviewed and updated frequently?

If using a search engine such as Google, Yahoo, or MSN Search, patients must be reminded that some web sites, often commercial, pay to be ranked near the top of some searches. This exposes patients to biased, commercial information.

Complementary and Alternative Medicines Commonly Used by People Living with Multiple Sclerosis

Biologically Based Therapies

Dietary Supplements

ANTIOXIDANTS

+ *Theory*: Free radicals may play a role in MS. Myelin may sustain injury by the free radicals released by immune cells. Oxidative damage may be involved in axonal damage. Antioxidants can decrease this damage.
+ *Risks*: Antioxidants may activate T cells and macrophages.
+ *Examples*: Vitamins A, C, and E; selenium; alpha-lipoic acid; inosine; uric acid; coenzyme Q10; grapeseed extract; pycnogenols; oligomeric proanthocyanidins (OPCs).

CRANBERRY

+ *Theory*: Cranberry products have been shown to inhibit UTIs by preventing bacteria from adhering to the bladder wall. In vitro, there is a mild antibiotic effect. Cranberry works best in women with normal bladder function.
+ *Risks*: Cranberry is not adequate to treat UTIs.
+ *Examples*: Cranberry tablets or extract. Small amounts of cranberry juice are not adequate to provide prevention.

ECHINACEA

+ *Theory*: Echinacea is widely used to prevent or shorten viral illnesses such as the common cold.
+ *Risks*: Limited studies have shown activation of T cells and macrophages involved in MS. This may have a detrimental effect on MS symptoms.
+ *Examples*: Other supplements that may boost immune system function include Asian ginseng, Siberian ginseng, garlic, antioxidants, zinc, and melatonin.

GINKGO BILOBA

+ *Theory*: Ginkgo biloba may have some value as an anti-inflammatory agent for use in MS but studies have not shown consistent benefit. The use of ginkgo biloba in the animal model of MS (experimental allergic encephalomyelitis [EAE]) and a small human study show effect on MS attacks. Another human study did not show this effect. Ginkgo may have some benefit in improving cognition in MS, but further studies are needed.

*   *Risks:* Ginkgo may cause thinning of the blood, and patients must be aware of this if they have bleeding disorders or are facing surgery. It may also increase seizures in people with seizures.

KAVA KAVA

*   *Theory:* Kava kava may reduce anxiety, mimicking the effects of benzo-diazepines.
*   *Risks:* Kava kava use has been associated with reports of severe liver toxicity. It is banned in Europe and Canada, but is available in the United States, with severe warnings. It is not felt to be adequate for severe anxiety. It may produce sedation, adding to MS fatigue.

ST. JOHN'S WORT

*   *Theory:* This botanical, used for centuries, has been shown in clinical trials to be effective for mild to moderate depression if taken in recommended amounts.
*   *Risks:* Depression can be serious; it should not be self-diagnosed and self-treated. St. John's Wort is not recommended for severe depression. It increases cytochrome P450, which may affect the metabolism of other medications.
*   *Examples:* Some "multivitamins for women" contain small amounts of St. John's wort.

VITAMIN B$_{12}$

*   *Theory:* Vitamin B$_{12}$ is essential for maintaining a healthy nervous system. In B$_{12}$ deficiency, patients may have injury to the optic nerves and spinal cord. Conclusions have been made that supplementation with B$_{12}$ will help in MS also.
*   *Risks:* Few.
*   *Examples:* Vitamin B$_{12}$, cobalamin, cyanocobalamin.

VITAMIN D AND CALCIUM

*   *Theory:* Vitamin D and calcium are important in maintaining bone density. People with MS may be more prone to osteopenia and osteoporosis due to inactivity, disability, and steroid use. Vitamin D may have a therapeutic effect on immune system function. Animal model studies of vitamin D showed an increased disease severity in EAE with Vitamin D deficiency, and improvement with supplementation of Vitamin D. Epidemiologic studies indicate that the use of Vitamin D supplements is associated with a decreased risk of developing MS.

+ *Risks:* Calcium may interfere with the absorption of some medications such as antibiotics, thyroid medications, and osteoporosis medication and minerals such as iron, magnesium, and zinc. Vitamin D and calcium in large amounts may cause multiple side effects.
+ Dietary calcium is more bioavailable, but supplements can be taken to reach the recommended daily allowance of 1,000 mg for those under 50 and 1,200 to 1,500 mg for those over 50.
+ *Examples:* Calcium citrate, calcium carbonate (both available with Vitamin D).

Diets

In general, based on scientific, epidemiologic, animal model, and clinical trial studies, diets that are low in saturated fats and high in polyunsaturated fatty acids (PUFAs) may have therapeutic effect in MS. PUFAs include omega-3 fatty acids (eicosapentaenoic acid [EPA], docosahexanoic acid [DHA], and alpha-linolenic acid [ALA]), and Omega-6 fatty acids (linoleic acid and gamma- linolenic acid).

THE SWANK DIET

+ *Theory:* Developed by Dr. Roy Swank during the 1940s, this diet was proposed based on epidemiologic studies that indicated MS was less common in populations that consume a diet low in saturated fats and high in levels of polyunsaturated fats (PUFAs). His diet was very low in saturated fats (15 g or less daily), excluded high-fat dairy products, and called for frequent fish meals, 10 to 15 g of vegetable oil and 5 g of cod liver oil daily. Benefits from the diet were shown to be fewer attacks, less progression of disability, and decreased mortality in people who were mildly affected by MS or who were early in the disease course.
+ *Risks:* Few risks exist for this diet. Protein amounts are low and must be monitored. Cod liver oil may have a blood thinning effect, and it does contain high levels of Vitamin A, which can be toxic in high doses.

OMEGA-6 FATTY ACIDS

+ *Theory:* Epidemiologic studies indicate that high consumption of PUFAs may be associated with a lower risk of developing MS. They may have anti-inflammatory and immune system modulating effects that, theoretically, could be therapeutic in MS. In animal models of MS, disease severity worsened with deficiencies of omega-6 and improved with supplementation. In human studies, results have not been consistent; however, in a re-analysis of data from several studies (some missing), the greatest effect seemed to be in mildly affected people; omege-6 fatty acids were not as beneficial in moderately or severely affected individuals. It is not effective in primary-progressive MS.

* *Risks:* Supplementation may cause vitamin E deficiency, which may need to be supplemented.
* *Examples:* Sunflower seed oil, evening primrose oil (has not shown therapeutic effects in people with relapsing-remitting or progressive disease), borage see ack t seed oil, and Spirulina (blue green algae).

OMEGA-3 FATTY ACIDS

* *Theory:* This approach is similar to that of omega-6 and the Swank diet. Studies have indicated that omega-3 fatty acids may have the most potent effect as an anti-inflammatory and immune modulator.
* *Risks:* Some fish, such as shark, swordfish, and king mackerel, contain high levels of mercury. Fish and flaxseed oils may have a blood thinning effect.
* *Examples:* Eicosapentaenoic acid (EPA) and docosahexanoic acid (DHA) are found in fatty fish such as salmon, Atlantic herring, Atlantic mackerel, blue fin tuna, and sardines. Dietary supplements containing DHA include fish oil and cod liver oil. Alpha-linolenic acid (ALA) is found in flaxseed oil, canola oil, and walnut oil.

BEE VENOM THERAPY

* *Theory:* This therapy involves inducing bees to sting the skin over affected areas, in the belief that the toxin will cause improvement in neurologic function. The theoretical explanation for this benefit is that bee toxin may an anti-inflammatory response, and chemical components of the venom may inhibit inflammatory proteins involved in MS. A component of bee venom, *apamin,* inhibits the effect of proteins on cells known as potassium channels (similar to effects of 4-aminopyridine). It is not known if the blood levels of bee venom are high enough to produce these effects.
* *Risks:* Bee venom could produce an anaphylactic reaction.

CANNABIS

* *Theory:* Cannabis (marijuana) can, theoretically, reduce symptoms of pain and spasticity in MS. The possibility exists that it can mildly suppress the immune system and protect against nerve cell injury.

♦ *Risks:* Smoking cannabis may cause nausea, vomiting, sedation, and increased seizures. It can impair driving ability for up to 8 hours. Chronic use may cause heart attacks, impair lung function, cause dependence and apathy, and increase the risk of cancers of the lung, head, and neck.
♦ *Examples:* Marijuana plant; also, prescription medications such as Marinol (U.S.) and Cesamet (Europe, Canada, and Australia).

HYPERBARIC OXYGEN

♦ *Theory:* Hyperbaric oxygen (HBO) involves breathing oxygen under increased pressure, thus increasing the amount of oxygen in blood and body tissues. It is accepted therapy for burns, severe infections, decompression sickness, radiation-induced tissue injury, and carbon monoxide poisoning. Many clinical trials have shown HBO to be ineffective in treating MS.
♦ *Risks:* Rare.

Alternative Medical Systems

ACUPUNCTURE AND TRADITIONAL CHINESE MEDICINE

♦ *Theory:* Traditional Chinese medicine utilizes methods that are designed to keep the energy of the body in balance and flowing. It utilizes many methods to do this including acupuncture, Chinese herbs, nutrition, exercise, stress reduction and massage. According to theory, disease occurs when disturbance or disharmony of energy is present. Acupuncture involves the insertion of thin needles into specific areas to alter the flow of energy to produce a therapeutic effect. Studies of the value of acupuncture in people with MS have been small, but it may provide benefit for bladder function, pain, nausea, and vomiting.
♦ *Risks:* Few, if done by a well-trained acupuncturist. Potential for infection exists.

Mind–Body Intervention

SPIRITUAL WELLNESS, MEDITATION, RELAXATION EXERCISES

♦ *Theory:* Patients who have a strong spiritual belief, practice meditation, or perform active relaxation exercises report benefit in restoring balance, decreasing stress, and in finding meaning and purpose. Spiritual wellness is not religion-specific, but rather encompasses the deeper meaning people feel in their lives from both within and possibly from belief in a higher power. Patients report, anecdotally, that they may feel less pain and emotional distress and possess a greater hope for the future.
♦ *Risks:* None.

Manipulative and Body-Based Therapies

CHIROPRACTIC MEDICINE

+ *Theory*: Chiropractic medicine is based on the belief that the nervous system plays a large role in physical health. Pressure from bones on the nerves in the spine that effect muscles and organs is thought to impair function. Practitioners of chiropractic medicine use manipulation techniques to adjust alignment of the spine to normalize bone positions and restore normal function. Many people living with MS utilize chiropractors. Although there are anecdotal reports of benefit for some symptoms, no studies have been conducted to look at the effect of chiropractic techniques on symptoms in MS or in altering the disease course. Chiropractic medicine should not be used in lieu of traditional medical care.
+ *Risks*: Few.

YOGA

+ *Theory*: Yoga exercises the mind, body, and spirit. Commonly, utilizing components of breathing, meditation, and posture, yoga may provide positive emotional benefits and physical benefits, such as increased strength and improved muscle stretch and balance. It can be adapted for people with MS and other disabilities.
+ *Risks*: Usually safe.

T'AI CHI

+ *Theory*: T'ai chi is a form of Chinese martial arts. It is believed to promote emotional balance, and it is also a form of exercise. It can improve balance, coordination, and increase strength. Studies are limited and inconclusive in MS, but it is widely practiced and can be adapted for people with disabilities.
+ *Risks*: T'ai chi is usually well tolerated.

MASSAGE

+ *Theory*: Massage is a form of body work that involves manipulation of soft tissue through pressure and traction. From a therapeutic view, it is thought to improve blood and lymph circulation, increase oxygen delivery, and remove toxins from the tissues. Anecdotally, it is reported to decrease spasticity for varying amounts of time. Massage is thought to release endorphins, which may promote mild pain relief. Patients report positive emotions from the touching aspect of massage.
+ *Risks*: Few.

Energy Therapies

STATIC MAGNETIC FIELD THERAPY

+ *Theory:* Some believe that disease can cause electrical imbalances within the body, which can be corrected with magnetic therapy. Anecdotally, people with MS report spasticity improvement, decreased pain, fatigue, improved bladder function, and improved quality of life. Studies of small, static, magnetic field therapies have been limited and report inconsistent findings. In the clinical setting, larger magnets used in pulsed fashion, have shown some benefit, especially with spasticity.
+ *Risks:* Few, but long-term use has not been studied.
+ *Examples:* Magnetized bracelets, insoles for shoes and mattresses.

Acknowledgment

I wish to thank Allen C. Bowling, M.D., Ph.D., for sharing his knowledge and mentoring me in my education about CAM. He pioneered this effort in the field of MS, and has been generous in providing material for this chapter.

REFERENCES

1. Sackett D, et al. Evidence-based medicine: what it is and what it isn't. *Br Med J.* 1996;7032:312.
2. Sackett D, et al. *Evidence-Based Medicine: How to Practice and Teach EBM.* New York: Churchill Livingstone; 2000:1.
3. Spiro H. Clinical reflections on the placebo phenomenon. In: Harrington A, ed. *The Placebo Effect.* Cambridge, MA: Harvard University Press, 1997.

Appendix: Additional Resources

Literature

Bowling AC. *Alternative Medicine and Multiple Sclerosis.* New York: Demos, 2001.

Bowling AC, Stewart TM. *Dietary Supplements and Multiple Sclerosis: A Health Professional's Guide.* New York: Demos, 2004.

Bowling AC, Ibrahim R, Stewart T. Alternative medicine and multiple sclerosis: an objective review from an American perspective. *Intern J MS Care.* 2000;2(3):14–21.

Health Canada. Facts about the Office of Natural Health Products and the Expert Advisory Committee on Natural Health Products (information booklet). March 1999.

Jellin JM, Batz F, Hitchens K. *Natural Medicines Comprehensive Database.*
    Stockton, CA: Therapeutic Research Faculty, 2005.

Polman CH, Thompson AJ, Murray TJ, et al. *Multiple Sclerosis: The Guide to
    Treatment and Management.* New York: Demos, 2006.

Sarubin-Fragakis A, American Dietetic Association. *The Health Professional's
    Guide to Popular Dietary Supplements,* 2nd ed. Chicago: American Dietetic
    Association, 2003.

Stewart TM, Bowling AC. Thinking about complementary and alternative
    medicine? An introduction for people with MS on how to find and evaluate claims
    about complementary and alternative medicine. MSAA, Cherry Hill, NJ:
    MSAA, 2006.

Web Sites

www.ms-cam.org. This site is maintained by the Rocky Mountain MS Center and
    contains MS-specific information about CAM therapies. Registration allows
    for participation in surveys to further research into CAM and MS.

nccam.nih.gov. This is an excellent starting point to learn about CAM in general,
    as well as to find information about particular CAM treatments.

www.fda.gov, www.cfsan.fda.gov, www.fda.gov/opacom/7alerts.html. The FDA is a
    good source of information about dietary supplements in particular.

www.ftc.gov, www.ftc.gov/bcp/menu-health.htm. The Federal Trade Commission is
    a good site to check on fraudulent claims or consumer alerts regarding a
    particular therapy.

www.nlm.nih.gov/nccam/camonpubmed.html. CAM on PubMed, maintained
    jointly by the NCCAM and the National Library of Medicine, provides
    access to peer-reviewed scientific articles on CAM therapies.

ods.od.nih.gov/databases/ibids.html. The International Bibliographic Information
    on Dietary Supplements (IBIDS) Database, maintained by the National
    Institute of Health Office of Dietary Supplements (ODS) provides access
    to peer-reviewed scientific articles.

CHAPTER 18

Dealing with Uncertainty: Sustaining Hope in Multiple Sclerosis

Linda A. Morgante

Moment by moment, we deal with uncertainty. Most of what we are uncertain about filters through our lives without much notice or concern. For example, will the weather be sunny for a particular outing, or will the traffic pose any obstacles on a busy day. More serious threats of uncertainty flooded our lives after September 11, 2001, and have left us wondering what will happen next. Few events, however, change our lives forever like the threat of an illness.

Uncertainty in illness can be an obstacle to hope because there is no assurance that the future will be something to look forward to. Many illnesses, such as cancer, HIV/AIDS, lupus, rheumatoid arthritis, heart disease, and diabetes share an uncertain course with multiple sclerosis (MS). This uncertainty, or unpredictability, pertains to how one feels on a day-to-day basis, as well as what the future holds for health, happiness, and peace of mind.

Uncertainty begins before the diagnosis of MS is confirmed. This is a period of terrible "fear of the unknown," a time when the body is experiencing new and often disturbing symptoms. With a confirmed diagnosis comes the reality that MS is a disease characterized by periods of stability, instability, and regained stability. A person with MS is never sure when a relapse will occur, what neurologic manifestations will be present, and what the outcome of the relapse will be. People with MS also deal with the day-to-day variability of myriad symptoms. Furthermore, the uncertainty of transitioning to a progressive course of MS can be a constant stressor for patients and their families. Nurses can help patients cope with uncertainty by shifting hope from its futuristic perspective to one of finding meaning in the experience and making the most of each day (1).

This chapter explores the concepts of uncertainty and hope in MS. It includes a review of the literature on uncertainty in illness, strategies for coping with uncertainty, and measures to keep hope alive for patients and families living with MS.

Review of the Literature: Uncertainty in Illness

Uncertainty is recognized as an important stressor in acute and chronic illness, one that often impairs quality of life. In the late 1980s, Mishel (2) proposed a theory to account for the uncertainty associated with the diagnosis, treatment, and recovery commonly experienced by people during acute illnesses. This theoretical framework proposed relationships among common aspects of the illness experience such as social support, symptom patterns, and relationships with healthcare providers, and the development and subsequent successful management of uncertainty. The theoretical framework also proposed a number of antecedents to uncertainty in illness, including illness severity, diagnostic specificity, personality factors, social support, healthcare providers, and patient demographics.

Several research studies conducted on various medical conditions affecting diverse patient populations have validated that uncertainty wanes over time, returns when illness recurs or exacerbates, and is highest during periods awaiting diagnosis (3). In acute illness, there is consistent and powerful evidence that uncertainty is associated with diminished quality of life (4). However, acute illnesses, even those that cause threats and consequences to a person's long-term health and well-being, are associated with some degree of closure, and these illnesses do not carry the continuous burden of uncertainty that is experienced in chronic illness.

In the early 1990s, Mishel (3) expanded her theory on uncertainty in illness to accommodate the ongoing uncertainty experienced by people living with chronic illness. This expanded theory proposed that uncertainty can be gradually accepted and integrated into one's life, rather than be managed or eliminated, as suggested in her previous work. Findings from studies across many chronic disease trajectories confirm that the unpredictability of disabling symptoms and lack of information about the future are important antecedents of long-term illness-related uncertainty. The studies also validate that personal growth and a changed view about life can emerge as successful consequences of coping with uncertainty over extended periods of time (4).

Uncertainty is very often described as a variable related to MS. Most articles written about MS mention uncertainty, or unpredictability, early on. In fact, most of the literature written for patients and families mention uncertainty as a phenomenon associated with living with the disease. In a recent study, Isaksson and Ahlstrom (5) described the emotional reactions of patients after the onset of the first symptoms and again following the MS diagnosis. Uncertainty emerged as a theme at both intervals. The uncertainty experienced before diagnosis was associated with not knowing what was wrong, and not receiving definitive answers or support from the healthcare providers. After receiving a conclusive diagnosis of MS, uncertainty focused on the prognosis and what the future would hold for that particular individual.

Miller (6) conducted a phenomenologic study of the lived experience of relapsing MS. In this study, uncertainty emerged as a theme for all the participants. Miller found that, because the disease is so unpredictable, her subjects did not know what to expect upon awakening each day. She also validated the notion that people are able to live one day at a time, hoping for the best.

Uncertainty and Hope

Uncertainty is often associated with hopelessness, powerlessness, frustration, and distress. Sallfors and colleagues (7) described this relationship in a qualitative study of children with juvenile chronic arthritis. The experience of chronic pain in the children sampled showed that living with this invisible symptom (similar to what people with MS describe) elicited emotional reactions that oscillated between hope and despair. Worry, anxiety, and suffering among the children were associated with living with uncertainty.

In another study, Morse and Penrod (8) looked at the relationship among the concepts of enduring, uncertainty, suffering, and hope in a number of groups of people experiencing an illness, injury, or a stressful life transition. The groups included individuals with spinal cord injuries, survivors of breast cancer, people awaiting heart transplants, and breast-feeding mothers who returned to work. Uncertainty was described as a state in which "the person knows where she or he wants to go but cannot identify how to get there. These people may have choice, but the course of each remains unknown and cannot be evaluated or compared. They do not have the information or the ability to weigh the odds nor to understand the alternatives. While they have no qualms about what they want as an outcome, the means to attain the goal remains unknown" (8; p. 148)." The authors state that uncertainty paralyzes hope, meaning the person is unable to select options or move ahead. "Despite the presence of a goal, the lack of a route does not enable the person to perceive the future as a reality, as an achievable option" (8; p.148). The authors conclude that "the state of uncertainty encompasses elements of enduring and suffering, rapidly moving between the two states. As a result, this state of uncertainty is characterized by emotional instability: the person endures the present and suffers the inability to envision a way out of the predicament; the person is suspended while hope is held in abeyance. Only with acknowledgment can the person move into suffering and through suffering and despair to hope" (8; p.149).

Wineman and colleagues (9) performed an analysis of the concepts of illness uncertainty, coping, hopefulness, and mood during participation in a clinical drug trial for MS. The authors found that people who experienced greater uncertainty and ambiguity about their MS were more likely to exhibit emotional distress, negative moods, and feel less hopefulness about the future.

The findings from these studies suggest that uncertainty and hope may have a cyclical relationship. They also demonstrate the extent of anguish and distress people living with uncertainty may experience. Discovering ways to help people through the uncertainty associated with MS is an important pathway to hope.

How Nurses Help Patients Cope with Uncertainty

The findings from the studies cited earlier provide clues to understanding how and when to help patients with MS cope with uncertainty. When patients experience the first onset of neurologic symptoms, they are frightened, and confused. Healthcare providers can add to the anxiety by not providing sufficient information and support. In the study by Isaksson and Ahlstrom (5), MS patients in the prediagnosis stage worried about what was wrong, viewed the experience as strange and unreal, and were confused by all that went into the experience of having a neurologic examination. In another study, the lack of information during this pre-diagnosis stage contributed to the fear that the symptoms were a manifestation of a terminal illness (10). Primary care providers and general neurology practices often do not have the resources or staff to spend time explaining and educating patients and families on what might possibly be the problem. A referral to a comprehensive MS care center can help to alleviate some of this uncertainty early on. At the center, a nurse often provides an explanation of what to expect, and clarifies other information for patients and families.

Support and kindness during this stage of the MS experience also help to alleviate the burden of uncertainty. Nurses are in a prime position to create an environment that is therapeutic by infusing it with empathy, unconditional positive regard, respect, warmth, and caring. It is clear that establishing a relationship and providing information and education to patients and families in the pre-diagnosis phase are keys to helping patients and families cope with uncertainty.

The diagnosis of MS is a time of recognition and acknowledgment that an illness exists. Although for some the diagnosis of MS comes as a relief that nothing is fatally wrong, the chronicity and unpredictability that accompany MS can create new fears and anxieties. In the era of treatment options for MS, uncertainty can be alleviated by the fact that medications are available to alter the natural history of the disease. These disease-modifying agents provide at least partial protection against exacerbations, and slow the progression of the illness for many people. But the available agents do not provide a guarantee that MS will never worsen for a particular individual.

Symptoms related to MS manifest differently in each person and change over time. Uncertainty is compounded by the day-to-day variability experienced by people with MS. For example, fatigue, a common symptom in MS, can worsen when the body's internal thermostat is elevated. Thus, on any given day, an individual who experiences MS-related fatigue may feel more tired if she has a fever, or the temperature outside is extremely hot. Planning each day, each moment, becomes a complicated task for people with MS, and adds to their overall uncertainty.

Education, counseling, disease-modifying treatment options, adequate management of symptoms, referrals to rehabilitative services, self-care strategies for promoting health and well-being (i.e., good nutrition, exercise, and stress-reducing techniques), ongoing support, guidance, and presence are some ways that nurses can help people cope with uncertainty throughout their life-long struggles with MS.

Keeping Hope Alive

"Hope is experiencing a sense of unlimited possibility and potential. It is a resource within each person that can be illuminated to promote healing" (1; p.213). People who live with uncertainty, with the unknown, are challenged to dig deep down inside to find meaning and possibility in the experience, so that they can feel hopeful. In this way, they can move past the boundaries of uncertainty to a new dimension and a new way of living life.

If uncertainty and hope are to exist together, then people must make choices about what will move them to a better place. The fears and anxieties that contribute to suffering must be managed, so that hope can become a reality. Nurses must be prepared for the fluctuations in the physical, cognitive, emotional, and spiritual distress that are just as much burdens of MS as the brain's lesion load. These fluctuations rekindle uncertainty and impede the hoping process. Good nursing care will ultimately bring a holistic, multidimensional approach that helps patients and families to make choices, deal with uncertainty, and keep hope alive.

Summary

Nurses share an intimate space with the patients and families whom they care for. Within this space, a person's search for meaning and making sense of an illness is guided by the nurse's energy, expertise, and well-spring of hope. In this space, healing can be an ongoing process, one that deals with the fluctuations of the MS experience. Nurses who care for people with MS can transform an uncertain experience into one of comfort and hope, helping patients deal with obstacles and threats in a realistic way, always clinging to the endless possibilities new research and treatments have to offer.

REFERENCES

1. Morgante L. Integrating the concept of hope into clinical practice. In: Halper J, Holland N, eds. *Comprehensive Nursing Care in Multiple Sclerosis*, 2nd ed. New York: Demos, 2002.

2. Mishel MH. Uncertainty in acute illness. In: Cohen FL, ed. *Annual Review of Nursing Research*, 15th ed. New York: Springer; 1997:57–80.

3. Mishel MH. Uncertainty in chronic illness. In: Fitzpatrick JJ, ed. *Annual Review of Nursing Research*, 17th ed. New York: Springer; 1999:269–294.

4. Brashers D, Neidig J, et al. The medical, personal, and social causes of uncertainty in HIV illness. *Issues Mental Health Nurs.* 2003;24:497–522.

5. Isaksson A, Ahlstrom G. From symptom to diagnosis: Illness experiences of multiple sclerosis patients. *J Neurosci Nurs.* 2006;38(4):229–237.

6. Miller C. The lived experience of relapsing multiple sclerosis: A phenomenological study. *J Neurosci Nurs.* 1997;29(5):294–304.

7. Sallfors C, Fasth A, Hallberg LR. Oscillating between hope and despair—a qualitative study. *Child Healthcare Dev.* 2002;28(6):495–505.

8. Morse J, Penrod J. Linking concepts of enduring, uncertainty, suffering, and hope. *Image J Nurs Scholarship.* 1999;31(2):145–150.

9. Weinman M, Schwetz K, et al. Longitudinal analysis of illness uncertainty, coping, hopefulness, and mood during participation in a clinical drug trial. *J Neurosci Nurs.* 2003;35(12):100–113.

10. Johnson J. On receiving the diagnosis of multiple sclerosis: Managing the transition. *Multiple Sclerosis.* 2003;9(1):82–88.

Resources

A vast array of resources is available to help you in your efforts to assist your patients with multiple sclerosis (MS). This list is by no means a complete one; it is designed as a starting point in your efforts to identify the resources you need to help your patients.

Recommended Reading

EKA Publications. *Guide to Catalogs for People with Disabilities, Their Families and Their Friends*. (EKA Publications, Inc., 9151 Hampton Overlook, Capital Heights, MD 20743; tel: 800-386-5367).

Gulick EE. Research priorities for nurses caring for persons with multiple sclerosis. Nursing Research Specialty Group of the Consortium of Multiple Sclerosis Centers. *J Neurosci Nurs.* 1996;28:314–321.

Halper J. The evolution of nursing care in multiple sclerosis. *Int J MS Care* [serial online]. 2000;3:13–20.

Halper J, Holland NJ, eds. *Comprehensive Nursing Care in Multiple Sclerosis*. New York: Demos, 1997.

Holland NJ, Halper J, eds. *Multiple Sclerosis: A Self-Care Guide to Wellness*. Washington DC: Paralyzed Veterans of America, 1998.

Medical Advisory Board NMSS. *Clinical Bulletin. Disease Management Consensus Statement.* New York: National Multiple Sclerosis Society, 1998.

Multiple Sclerosis in 1998. Continuing Education Program, National Multiple Sclerosis Society, Consortium of Multiple Sclerosis Centers, 1998.

Multiple Sclerosis: Key Issues in Nursing Management. New York: Bioscience. 2004.

Multiple Sclerosis—Challenges and Consensus. Continuing Education Program. Physicians World Communications, 1998.

Muma RD, Lyons BA, et al. *Patient Education: A Practical Approach.* Stamford CT: Appleton & Lange, 1996.

Parenting with a Disability. (Through the Looking Glass, 2198 Sixth Street, Suite 100, Berkeley, CA 94710; tel: 510-848-1112; 800-644-2666; www.lookingglass.org).

Peterman Schwarz S. *Dressing Tips and Clothing Resources for Making Life Easier.* Real Living with MS, 1111 Bethlehem Pike, P.O. Box 908, Springhouse, PA 19477).

Polman CH, Thompson AJ, Murray TJ, McDonald WI. *Multiple Sclerosis: The Guide to Treatment and Management,* 5th ed. Demos Medical Publishing, New York, 2001.

Rankin SH, Stallings KD. *Patient Education: Issues, Principles, Practices,* 2nd ed. Philadelphia: Lippincott, 1990.

Additional Reading

Avonex® Biogen Idec. Available at: http://www.avonex.com. Accessed December 2006.

BETA Nurse Program. Available at: www.mspathways.com. Accessed August 2006.

Burden M. Diabetes: treatment and complications- the nurse's role. *Nurs Times* 2003;99 (2):30–.32.

Clanet M, et al. Results of the European interferon beta 1-a (Avonex) dose-comparison study. *J Neurol* 2001;248(Suppl 2):A148.

Cohen JA, et al. Results of IMPACT, a Phase 3 trial of interferon beta-1a in secondary progressive MS. *Neurology* 2001;56(Suppl 3):A148–A149.

Comi G, et al. Effect of early interferon treatment on conversion to definite multiple sclerosis: a randomised study. *Lancet* 2001;357(9268):1576–1582.

Comi G, et al. European/Canadian multicenter, double-blind, randomized, placebo-controlled study of the effects of glatiramer acetate on magnetic resonance imaging–measured disease activity and burden in patients with relapsing multiple sclerosis. European/Canadian Glatiramer Acetate Study Group. *Ann Neurol* 2001;49(3):290–297.

Copaxone® Teva Pharmaceutical Industries Ltd. Available at: http://www.mswatch.com/. Accessed December 2006.

Denis L, et al. Long-term treatment optimization in individuals with multiple sclerosis using disease-modifying therapies: a nursing approach. *J Neurosci Nurs* 2004;36(1):10–22.

Dhib-Jalbut S. Mechanisms of action of interferons and glatiramer acetate in multiple sclerosis. *Neurology* 2002;58(8 Suppl 4):S3–S9.

Funnell MM, et al. Self-management support for insulin therapy in type 2 diabetes. *Diabetes Educ* 2004;30(2):274–280.

Goodin DS, et al. Disease modifying therapies in multiple sclerosis: report of the Therapeutics and Technology Assessment Subcommittee of the American Academy of Neurology and the MS Council for Clinical Practice Guidelines. *Neurology* 2002;58(2):169–178.

Goodkin DE, et al. The North American Study of interferon beta-1b in secondary progressive multiple sclerosis. 52nd Annual Meeting of the American Academy of Nuerology, San Diego, CA. 2000: Abstract #LBN.002.

Halper J. Role of advanced practise nurse in management of multiple sclerosis. *Int J MS Care* 2006;8:33–38.

Holland NJ, et al. Nursing grand rounds: multiple sclerosis. *J Neurosci Nurs* 2005;37(1):15–19.

Interferon beta-1b in the treatment of multiple sclerosis: final outcome of the randomized controlled trial. The IFNB Multiple Sclerosis Study Group and The University of British Columbia MS/MRI Analysis Group. *Neurology* 1995;45(7):1277–1285.

Interferon beta-1b is effective in relapsing-remitting multiple sclerosis. I. Clinical results of a multicenter, randomized, double-blind, placebo-controlled trial. The IFNB Multiple Sclerosis Study Group. *Neurology* 1993;43(4):655–661.

International Organizations of Multiple Sclerosis Nurses. Available at: http://www.iomsn.org. Accessed December 2006.

Jacobs LD, et al. Intramuscular interferon beta-1a for disease progression in relapsing multiple sclerosis. The Multiple Sclerosis Collaborative Research Group (MSCRG). *Ann Neurol* 1996;39(3):285–294.

Jacobs LD, et al. Intramuscular interferon beta-1a therapy initiated during a first demyelinating event in multiple sclerosis. CHAMPS Study Group. *N Engl J Med* 2000;343(13):898–904.

Johnson KP, et al. Copolymer 1 reduces relapse rate and improves disability in relapsing-remitting multiple sclerosis: results of a Phase III multicenter, double-blind placebo-controlled trial. The Copolymer 1 Multiple Sclerosis Study Group. *Neurology* 1995;45(7):1268–1276.

Kappos L, et al. Treatment with interferon beta-1b delays conversion to clinically definite and McDonald MS in patients with clinically isolated syndromes. *Neurology* 2006;67(7):1242–1249.

Li DK, et al. Magnetic resonance imaging results of the PRISMS trial: a randomized, double-blind, placebo-controlled study of interferon-beta1a in relapsing-remitting multiple sclerosis. Prevention of Relapses and Disability by Interferon-beta1a Subcutaneously in Multiple Sclerosis. *Ann Neurol* 1999;46(2):197–206.

Li DK, et al. Randomized controlled trial of interferon-beta-1a in secondary progressive MS: MRI results. *Neurology* 2001;56(11):1505–1513.

Long AF, et al. The role of the nurse within the multi-professional rehabilitation team. *J Adv Nurs* 2002;37(1):70–78.

Lublin FD, et al. Effect of relapses on development of residual deficit in multiple sclerosis. *Neurology* 2003;61(11):1528–1532.

Lublin FD. History of modern multiple sclerosis therapy. *J Neurol* 2005; 252(Suppl 3):3–9.

Madonna MG, et al. Multiple sclerosis pathways: an innovative nursing role in disease management. *J Neurosci Nurs* 1999;31(6):332–335.

National multiple sclerosis society. Available at: http://www.nationalmssociety. org. Accessed December 2006.

Newbold D. Coping with rheumatoid arthritis. How can specialist nurses influence it and promote better outcomes? *J Clin Nurs* 1996; 5(6):373–380.

Newbold D. Health economics and nursing management. *J Nurs Manag* 2005; 13(5):373–376.

Novantrone® Serono, Inc. Prescribing information. Available at: http://www. novantrone.com/assets/pdf/novantrone_prescribing_info.pdf. Accessed August 2006.

Paty DW, et al. Interferon beta-1b is effective in relapsing-remitting multiple sclerosis. II. MRI analysis results of a multicenter, randomized, double-blind, placebo-controlled trial. UBC MS/MRI Study Group and the IFNB Multiple Sclerosis Study Group. *Neurology* 1993;43(4):662–667.

Paty DW, et al. Interferon beta-lb is effective in relapsing-remitting multiple sclerosis. II. MRI analysis results of a multicenter, randomized, double-blind, placebo-controlled trial. *Neurology* 2001;57(12 Suppl 5):S10–S15.

Placebo-controlled multicentre randomised trial of interferon beta-1b in treatment of secondary progressive multiple sclerosis. European Study Group on interferon beta-1b in secondary progressive MS. *Lancet* 1998; 352(9139):1491–1497.

Porter B, et al. Nursing at a specialist diagnostic clinic for multiple sclerosis. *Br J Nurs* 2003;12(11):650, 652–656.

PRISMS. PRISMS-4: long-term efficacy of interferon-beta-1a in relapsing MS. *Neurology* 2001;56(12):1628–1636.

PRISMS. Randomised double-blind placebo-controlled study of interferon beta-1a in relapsing/remitting multiple sclerosis. PRISMS (Prevention of Relapses and Disability by Interferon beta-1a Subcutaneously in Multiple Sclerosis) Study Group. *Lancet* 1998;352(9139):1498–1504.

Rebif® Serono Inc. and Pfizer Inc. Available at: http://www.mslifelines.com/ index.jsp. Accessed December 2006.

Rieckmann P. Neurodegeneration and clinical relevance for early treatment in multiple sclerosis. *Int MS J* 2005;12(2):42–51.

Rizvi SA, et al. Current approved options for treating patients with multiple sclerosis. *Neurology* 2004;63(12 Suppl 6):S8–S14.

Rudick RA, et al. Impact of interferon beta-1a on neurologic disability in relapsing multiple sclerosis. The Multiple Sclerosis Collaborative Research Group (MSCRG). *Neurology* 1997;49(2):358–363.

Scanzillo J, et al. Product enhancements decrease the incidence of injection site reactions and pain improving adherence to therapy in patients with multiple sclerosis. 22nd Congress of the European Committee for Treatment and Research in Multiple Sclerosis; September 27–30, 2006; Madrid, Spain. 2006.

Shapiro R. Adherence to interferon beta-1b: BETA Nurse program. 2005.

Simon JH, et al. Magnetic resonance studies of intramuscular interferon beta-1a for relapsing multiple sclerosis. The Multiple Sclerosis Collaborative Research Group. *Ann Neurol* 1998;43(1):79–87.

SPECTRIMS. Randomized controlled trial of interferon-beta-1a in secondary progressive MS: clinical results. *Neurology* 2001;56(11):1496–1504.

The MS Information Source Book. Available at: http://www.nationalmssociety.org/Sourcebook-Cognitive.asp. Accessed November 2006.

Thompson AJ, et al. Diagnostic criteria for primary progressive multiple sclerosis: a position paper. *Ann Neurol* 2000;47(6):831–835.

Thompson DM, et al. Insulin adjustment by a diabetes nurse educator improves glucose control in insulin-requiring diabetic patients: a randomized trial. *CMAJ* 1999;161(8):959–962.

Tysabri® Serono, Inc. Prescribing information. Available at: http://www.tysabri.com/downloads/product_information.pdf. Accessed 30 Aug 2006.

US Food and Drug Administration website/ Center for Drug Evaluation and Research. Available at: http://www.fda.gov/cder/drug/infopage/natalizumab/. Accessed December 2006.

Vajda FJ. Neuroprotection and neurodegenerative disease. *J Clin Neurosci* 2002; 9(1):4–8.

Warner R, et al. Improving service delivery for relapse management in multiple sclerosis. *Br J Nurs* 2005;14(14):746–753.

Yong VW. Differential mechanisms of action of interferon-beta and glatiramer aetate in MS. *Neurology* 2002;59(6):802–808.

Ziemssen T. Neuroprotection and glatiramer acetate: the possible role in the treatment of multiple sclerosis. *Adv Exp Med Biol* 2004;541:111–134.

Resource Materials

Assistive Technology Sourcebook. (Written by A. Enders and M. Hall, published by Resna Press, Washington, DC 1990.)

The Complete Directory for People with Disabilities, 1999–2000. (Published by Grey House Publishing, Inc., Pocket Knife Square, P.O. Box 1866, Lakeville, CT 06039; tel: 800-562-2139; fax: 860-435-3004; e-mail: www.greyhouse.com.)

Complete Drug Reference. (Compiled by United States Pharmacopoeia, published by Consumer Report Books, A division of Consumers Union, Yonkers, NY). This comprehensive, readable, and easy-to-use drug reference includes almost every prescription and nonprescription medication available in the United States and Canada. A new edition is published yearly.

Directory of National Information Sources on Disabilities. (Published by the National Institute on Disability and Rehabilitation Research, Washington, DC 1994–1995. Vols. I and II.)

Exceptional Parent: Parenting Your Child or Young Adult with a Disability. A magazine for families and professionals. (Exceptional Parent, P.O. Box 3000, Dept. EP, Denville, NJ 07834, tel: 800-247-8080.) A monthly magazine that celebrated its 25th anniversary by producing the *1996 Resource Guide*, which includes 10 directories with more than 1,000 resources in the United States and Canada. This is a very useful directory for adults with disabilities as well.

Living with Low Vision: A Resource Guide for People with Sight Loss. (Resources for Rehabilitation, 33 Bedford Street, Suite 19A, Lexington, MA 02173, tel: 617-862-6455.) The only large-print comprehensive guide to services and products designed to assist individuals with vision loss throughout North America.

Resources for People with Disabilities and Chronic Conditions. (Resources for Rehabilitation, 33 Bedford Street, Suite 19A, Lexington, MA 02173, tel: 617-862-6455.) A comprehensive resource guide covering a variety of disabling conditions as well as general information on rehabilitation services, assistive technology for independent living, and laws that affect people with disabilities.

Shrout RN. Resource Directory for the Disabled. New York: Facts-on-File, 1991. (Facts on File, 460 Park Avenue South, New York, NY 10016.) A resource directory that includes associations and organizations, government agencies, libraries and research centers, publications, and products of all types for disabled individuals.

Nursing Organizations

American Academy of Nurse Practitioners (Capitol Station LBJ Bldg., P.O. Box 12846, Austin, TX 78711, tel: 202-463-6930); American College of Nurse Practitioners (2401 Pennsylvania Avenue N.W., Suite 900, Washington, DC 20006, tel: 202-466-4825); National Alliance of Nurse Practitioners (325 Pennsylvania Avenue S.E., Washington, DC 2003, tel: 202-675-6350). Three national organizations representing nurse practitioners. Activities include legislative awareness, advocacy, professional education, and certification and/or recognition of advanced practice nurses.

American Association of Neuroscience Nurses (224 N. Des Plaines, Suite 60, Chicago, IL 60661, tel: 312-993-0043). This organization focuses on neurologic and neurosurgical conditions and techniques, both nursing and technological, which enhance patients' quality of life and survival. Annual meetings and a professional journal are offered to members and interested nurses.

American Association of Spinal Cord Injury Nurses (AASCIN) (75-20 Astoria Blvd., Jackson Heights, NY 11370-1177, tel: 718-803-3782). Although its focus is on spinal cord injury, this organization focuses on research and education with many concerns common to multiple sclerosis.

American Nurses Association (8515 Georgia Avenue, Silver Spring MD 20910). A national organization for nurses that offers a wide array of educational, research, and legislative services. In addition, ANCC, a branch of ANA, offers opportunities for certification in nursing specialties.

American Society of Neurorehabilitation (2221 University Avenue S.E., Suite 360, Minneapolis, MN 55414, tel: 612-623-2405). ASNR's membership consists of physicians and nonphysicians whose practice is devoted to patients with neurologic disease. ASNR publishes a journal, has an annual meeting, and holds certification courses for specialists.

Association of Rehabilitation Nurses (ARN) (5700 Old Orchard Road, 1st floor, Skokie, IL 60077-1057, tel: 708-966-3433). The ARN is an international organization of professional rehabilitation nurses. ARN offers a wide range of professional activities that help develop the professional skills of rehabilitation nurses. Included in these are educational conferences, seminars throughout the year, certification examinations, and support of research.

Nurse Practitioner Associates for Continuing Education (NPACE) (5 Militia Drive, Lexington, MA 02173, tel: 617-861-0270). NPACE conducts educational seminars for advanced practice nurses throughout the year.

Respiratory Nursing Society (RNS) (5700 Old Orchard Road, 1st floor, Skokie, IL 60077-1057, tel: 708-966-3433). RNS is the professional association for nurses who care for clients with pulmonary dysfunction and who are interested in the promotion of pulmonary health.

The Society of Urologic Nurses and Associates (E. Holly Avenue, Box 56, Pitman, NJ 08071-0056). A specialty group of nurses with a focus on urologic management problems.

Visiting Nurse Associations of America (VNAA) (3801 East Florida Avenue, Suite 900, Denver, CO 80210, tel: 800-426-2547). VNAA is a national, nonprofit, community-based organization of home healthcare providers.

Medical Organizations

American Academy of Neurology (2221 University Avenue S.E., Suite 335, Minneapolis, MN 55414, tel: 612-623-8115). Representing neurologists throughout North America, the AAN has recently established new membership criteria for nurses who specialize in care of the neurologically impaired patient.

American Neurologic Association (5841 Cedar Lake Road, #108, Minneapolis, MN 55416, tel: 612-545-6284.) The ANA offers membership to neurologists with an academic emphasis.

Multiple Sclerosis Organizations

National Multiple Sclerosis Society (NMSS) (733 Third Avenue, New York, NY 10017, tel: 800-FIGHT MS). The NMSS funds both basic and health services research. An office of professional education programs maintains a speakers' bureau and supports professional education programs in the individual chapters. Chapters and branches of the Society provide direct services to people with MS and their families, including information and referral, counseling, equipment loan, and social and recreational support programs. The National Office will put you in touch with your closest chapter. The Information Center and Library is available to answer questions and provide a wide range of educational materials, as well as reprints of articles written about MS.

Multiple Sclerosis Association of America (706 Haddonfield Road, Cherry Hill, NJ 08002 www.msaa.org). A national organization that provides patients with publications, equipment, educational programs, and services as the MRI Institute.

Multiple Sclerosis Society of Canada (250 Bloor Street East, Suite 820, Toronto, Ontario M4W 3P9, Canada, tel: 416-922-6065; in Canada: 800-268-7582). A national organization that funds research, promotes public education, and produces publications in both English and French. They provide an "ASK MS Information System" database of articles on a wide variety of topics including treatment, research, and social services. Regional divisions and chapters are located throughout Canada.

Multiple Sclerosis Foundation (6350 N. Andrews Avenue, Ft. Lauderdale, FL 33309 www.msf.org). A national organization providing patients and healthcare professionals with special services and unique educational programs.

Electronic Information Sources

One of the most flexible ways to obtain information on MS is online. Many sources of information are available free through the Internet, on the World Wide Web. For example, the National Multiple Sclerosis Society has a home page on the World Wide Web at: http://www.nmss.org/. If you are an experienced "net surfer," switch to your favorite search facility and enter the key words "MS" or "multiple sclerosis." This generally will give you a listing of dozens of web sites that pertain to MS. Keep in mind, however, that the World Wide Web is a free and open medium; while many of the web sites have excellent and useful information, others may contain highly unusual and inaccurate information.

The following web sites are especially good sources of information.

MS-Specific Organizations

International Organization of MS Nurses
http://www.iomsn.org

The Consortium of Multiple Sclerosis Centers
http://www.mscare.org/

CLAMS—Computer Literate Advocates for Multiple Sclerosis
http://www.clams.org/

Multiple Sclerosis International Foundation
http://www.msif.org

The International Journal of MS Care
http://www.mscare.com/

The Multiple Sclerosis Information Gateway
Schering AG, Berlin, Germany
http://www.ms-gateway.com/

The Multiple Sclerosis Society of Canada
http://www.mssoc.ca/

The National Multiple Sclerosis Society
http://www.nmss.org/

Multiple Sclerosis Society of Canada
http://mssociety.ca

Understanding MS
http://www.understandingms.com

MS Watch
http://www.mswatch.com

Computer Literate Advocates for MS (CLAMS)
http://www.clams.org

Healthfinder
http://www.healthfinder.gov

MSwatch
http://www.mswatch.com

Caregiving Online
www.caregiving.com

Nursing Home Abuse and Neglect
http://www.txlegal.com/nursing.htm

Multiple Sclerosis Trust
http://www.mstrust.org.uk

Multiple sclerosis Society of UK
http://www.mssociety.org.uk

Web MD Health
http://www.webmd.com

NIH National Center for Complementary and Alternative Medicine
http://www.nccam.nih.gov

National Academy of Neuropsychology
http://nanonline.org

Pharmaceutical Company Websites

Serono Inc./Rebif
http://www.serono.com/ms/

Berlex/Betaseron
http://www.betaseron.com/

Biogen/Idec/Avonex Tysabri
http://www.biogen.com/

Teva Neuroscience/Copaxone
http://www.tevaneuro.com/

Genentech/Rituximab
http://www.genentech.com

Novartis
http://www.novartis.com

General Interest

ABLEDATA
Information on assistive technology
http://www.abledata.com/

Allsup, Inc
Assists individuals applying for Social Security disability benefits
http://www.allsupinc.com/

Apple Computer Disability Resources
http://www.apple.com/education/k12/disability/

CenterWatch Clinical Trials Listing Service™
http://www.centerwatch.com/

IBM Special Needs Systems
http://www.austin.ibm.com/sns/

Infosci
Selected links on MS
http://www.infosci.org/

Medicare Information
http://www.hcfa.gov/medicare/medicare.htm

Microsoft Accessibility Technology for Everyone
http://www.microsoft.com/enable/

The National Family Caregivers Association
http://www.nfcacares.org/

The National Institute of Neurological Disorders and Stroke
http://www.ninds.nih.gov/

The National Library of Medicine
http://www.nlm.nih.gov/

The National Organization for Rare Disorders
http://www.rarediseases.org/

NARIC—The National Rehabilitation Information Center
http://www.naric.com/

Information Sources on Disability-Related Issues

Accent on Information (P.O. Box 700, Bloomington, IL 61702, tel: 304-378-2961). A computerized retrieval system of information for the disabled about problems relating to activities of daily living and home management. There is a small charge for a basic search and photocopies, but disabled persons unable to pay are never denied services.

Canadian Rehabilitation Council for the Disabled (CRCD) (45 Sheppard Avenue East, Suite 801, Toronto, Ontario M2N 5W9, Canada, tel: 416-250-7490). The Council is a federation of regional and provincial groups serving individuals with disabilities throughout Canada. It operates an information service and publishes a newsletter and a quarterly journal.

Clearinghouse on Disability Information (Office of Special Education and Rehabilitative Services, U.S. Department of Education, Switzer Building, 330 C Street, S.W., Washington, DC 20202, tel: 202-205-8241). Created by the Rehabilitation Act of 1973, the Clearinghouse responds to inquiries about federal laws, services, and programs for individuals of all ages with disabilities. Their quarterly magazine, *OSERS News in Print*, is available free of charge.

Disability Rights Center (1616 P Street, N.W., Suite 435, Washington, DC 20036, tel: 202-328-5198). The DIRS provides information about services available to people with disabilities and their families. Through its computerized database, DIRS provides information from both the public and the private sectors.

Information Center and Library, National Multiple Sclerosis Society (733 Third Avenue, New York, NY 10017, tel: 800-FIGHT MS). The Center will answer questions and send you publications of the Society as well as copies of published articles on any topics related to MS.

Inglis House (2600 Belmont Avenue, Philadelphia, PA 19131, tel: 215-878-5600). A national information exchange network specializing in long-term facilities for mentally alert people with physical disabilities.

National Health Information Center (P.O. Box 1133, Washington, DC 20013, tel: 800-336-4797). The Center maintains a library and a database of health-related organizations. It also provides referrals related to health issues for consumers and professionals.

President's Committee on Employment of the Handicapped (1111 20th Street N.W. 6th floor, Washington, DC 20036, tel: 202-635-5010). The President's Committee publishes and distributes free pamphlets, publications, and posters covering such topics as education, employment, accessibility, and adapting the worksite. The Committee also publishes *Disabled USA*.

Rehabilitation Research Institute (Academic Center T-605, George Washington University, Washington, DC 20502, tel: 202-676-2624). The Institute develops and disseminates materials for rehabilitation professions and the general public. Publications include annotated bibliographies and covers topics such as attitudinal barriers, employment rights, recreation, and sexual disability.

Agencies and Organizations

American Self-Help Clearinghouse (St. Clares–Riverside Medical Center, Denville, NJ 07834, tel: 201-625-7101). The Clearinghouse makes referrals to national self-help organizations as well as individual self-help groups for various problems. They also provide referrals to local self-help clearinghouses.

Beach Center on Families and Disabilities (c/o Life Span Institute, University of Kansas, 3111 Haworth Hall, Lawrence, KS 66045, tel: 913-864-7600). The federally funded Center conducts research and training about the functioning of families in which one member is disabled. They have a publications catalog relating to family coping, professional roles, and service delivery. They offer a free newsletter, "Families and Disability."

Consortium of Multiple Sclerosis Centers (CMSC) (c/o MS Center at Holy Name Hospital, 718 Teaneck Road, Teaneck, NJ 07666, tel: 201-837-0727). The CMSC is made up of numerous MS centers throughout the United States and Canada. The Consortium's mission is to disseminate information to clinicians, increase resources and opportunities for research, and advance the standard of care for multiple sclerosis. The CMSC is a multidisciplinary organization, bringing together healthcare professionals from many fields involved in MS patient care.

Department of Veterans Affairs (VA) (810 Vermont Avenue, N.W., Washington, DC 20420, tel: 202-328-5198). The VA provides a wide range of benefits and services to those who have served in the armed forces, their dependents, beneficiaries of deceased veterans, and dependent children of veterans with severe disabilities.

Equal Employment Opportunity Commission (EEOC) (1801 L Street, N.W., 10th floor, Washington, DC 20507, tel: 800-669-3362 (to order publications); 800-669-4000 (to speak to an investigator; 202-663-4900). The EEOC is responsible for monitoring the section of the ADA on employment regulations. Copies of the regulations are available.

Handicapped Organized Women (HOW) (P.O. Box 35481, Charlotte, NC 28235, tel: 704-376-4735). HOW strives to build self-esteem and confidence among disabled women by encouraging volunteer community involvement. HOW seeks to train disabled women for leadership positions and works in conjunction with the National Organization of Women (NOW).

Health Resource Center for Women with Disabilities (Rehabilitation Institute of Chicago, Chicago, IL 60612, tel: 312-908-7997). The Center is a project run by and for women with disabilities. It publishes a free newsletter, "Resourceful Women," and offers support groups and educational seminars addressing issues from a disabled woman's perspective. Among its many educational resources, the Center has developed a video on mothering with a disability.

National Council on Disability (NCOD) (800 Independence Avenue, S.W., Suite 814, Washington, DC 20591, tel: 202-267-3846). The Council is an independent federal agency whose role is to study and make recommendations about public policy for people with disabilities. Publishes a free newsletter, "Focus."

National Family Caregivers Association (NFCA) (9621 East Bexhill Drive, Kensington, MD 20895, tel: 301-942-6430). NFCA is dedicated to improving the quality of life of America's 18,000,000 caregivers. It publishes a quarterly newsletter, and has a resource guide, an information clearinghouse, and a toll-free hotline: 800-896-3650.

Office on the Americans with Disabilities Act (Department of Justice, Civil Rights Division, P.O. Box 66118, Washington, DC 20035, tel: 202-514-0301). This office is responsible for enforcing the ADA. To order copies of its regulations, call 202-514-6193.

Paralyzed Veterans of America (PVA) (801 Eighteenth Street N.W., Washington, DC20006, tel: 800-424-8200). PVA is a national information and advocacy agency working to restore function and quality of life for veterans with spinal cord dysfunction. It supports and funds education and research and has a national advocacy program that focuses on accessibility issues. PVA publishes brochures on many issues related to rehabilitation.

President's Committee on Employment of People with Disabilities (1331 F Street, N.W., Washington, DC 20004-1107; tel: 202-376-6200; Internet: www.info@pcepd.gov). The Committee publishes employment-related brochures for individuals with disabilities and their employers, and provides the Job Accommodation Network (tel: 800-526-7234).

Social Security Administration (6401 Security Boulevard, Baltimore, MD 21235, tel: 800-772-1213). To apply for social security benefits based on disability, call this office or visit your local social security branch office. The Office of Disability within the Social Security Administration publishes a free brochure entitled, "Social Security Regulations: Rules for Determining Disability and Blindness."

United Spinal Association (75-20 Astoria Boulevard, Jackson Heights, NY 11370, tel: 718-803-EPVA). United Spinal Association is a private, nonprofit organization dedicated to serving the needs of its members as well as other people with disabilities. While offering a wide range of benefits to member veterans with spinal cord dysfunction (including hospital liaison, sports and recreation, wheelchair repair, adaptive architectural consultations, research and educational services, communications, and library and information services), they will also provide brochures and information on a variety of subjects, free of charge to the general public.

Well Spouse Foundation (P.O. Box 801, New York, NY 10023, tel: 212-724-7209). An emotional support network for people married to or living with a chronically ill partner. Advocacy for home health and long-term care and a newsletter are among the services offered.

Assistive Technology

ABLEDATA (8455 Colesville Road Suite 935, Silver Spring, MD 20910, tel: 301;588-9284; 800-227-0216; fax: 301-589-3563. ABLEDATA is a national database of information on assistive technology designed to enable persons with disabilities to identify and locate the devices that will assist them in their home, work, and leisure activities. Information specialists are available to answer questions during regular business hours. ABLE INFORM BBS is available twenty-four hours a day to customers with a computer, modem, and telecommunications software.

Access to Recreation: Adaptive Recreation Equipment for the Physically Challenged (2509 E. Thousand Oaks Boulevard, Suite 430, Thousand Oaks, CA 91362, tel: 800-634-4351). Products include exercise equipment and assistive devices for sports, environmental access, games, crafts, and hobbies.

adaptABILITY (Department 2082, Norwich Avenue, Colchester, CT 06415, tel: 800-243-9232). A free catalog of assistive devices and self-care equipment designed to enhance independence.

American Automobile Association (1712 G Street N.W., Washington, DC 20015). The AAA will provide a list of automobile hand-control manufacturers.

AT&T Special Needs Center (2001 Route 46, Parsippany, NJ 07054, tel: 800-233-1222). A catalog of special telephone equipment for individual with physical disabilities.

Enrichments (P.O. Box 5050, Bolingbrook, IL 60440, tel: 800-323-5547). A free catalog of assistive devices and self-care equipment designed to enhance independence.

Medic Alert Foundation International (P.O. Box 1009, Turlock, CA 95380, tel: 800-344-3226; 209-668-3333). A medical identification tag worn to identify a person's medical condition, medications, and any other important information that might be needed in case of an emergency. A file of the person's health data is maintained in a central database to be accessed by a physician or other emergency personnel who need to know the person's pertinent medical information.

National Rehabilitation Information Center (NARIC) (8455 Colesville Road, Silver Spring, MD 20910, tel: 800-346-2742; 301-588-9284; fax: 301-587-1967). NARIC is a library and information center on disability and rehabilitation, funded by the National Institute on Disability and Rehabilitation Research (NIDRR). NARIC operates two databases—ABLEDATA and REHABDATA. NARIC collects and disseminates the results of federally funded research projects and has a collection that includes commercially published books, journal articles, and audiovisual materials. NARIC is committed to serving both professionals and consumers who are interested in disability and rehabilitation. Information specialists can answer simple information requests and provide referrals immediately and at no cost. More complex database searches are available at nominal cost.

REHABDATA (8455 Colesville Road, Suite 935, Silver Spring, MD 20910, tel: 301-588-9284; 800-346-2742) REHABDATA is a database containing bibliographic records with abstracts and summaries of the materials contained in the NARIC (National Rehabilitation Information Center) library of disability rehabilitation materials. Information specialists are available to conduct a database search on any rehabilitation related topic.

RESNA (1101 Connecticut Avenue N.W., Suite 700, Washington, DC 20036, tel: 202-857-1199). RESNA is an international association for the advancement of rehabilitation technology. Their objectives are to improve the quality of life for the disabled through the application of science and technology and to influence policy relating to the delivery of technology to disabled persons. They will respond by mail to specific questions about modifying existing equipment and designing new devices.

Sears Home Healthcare Catalog (P.O. Box 3123, Naperville, IL 60566, tel: 800-326-1750). The catalog includes medical equipment such as hospital beds, commodes, and wheelchairs, as well as adaptive clothing.

Sentry Detection Corporation (exclusive Westinghouse distributor) (tel: 800-695-0110). The company will install a Life Alert system (separately or as part of a total home security system) that allows a disabled person to get immediate assistance in the event of an emergency.

Environmental Adaptations

A Consumer's Guide to Home Adaptation (Adaptive Environments Center, 374 Congress Street, Suite 301, Boston, MA 02210, tel: 617-695-1225). A workbook for planning adaptive. home modifications such as lowering kitchen countertops and widening doorways.

"Adapting the Home for the Physically Challenged" (A/V Health Services, P.O. Box 1622, West Sacramento, CA 95691, tel: 703-389-4339). A 22-minute videotape that describes home modifications for individuals who use walkers or wheelchairs. Ramp construction and room modification specifications are included.

American Institute of Architects (AIA) (1735 New York Avenue, N.W., Washington, DC 20006, tel: 800-365-2724; publications catalog and orders: 202- 626-7300). This organization will make referrals to architects who are familiar with the design requirements of people with disabilities.

Barrier-Free Design Centre (2075 Bayview Avenue, Toronto, Ontario M4N 3M5, Canada, tel: 416-480-6000). The Centre provides information and technical consultation in barrier-free design for Canadians with physical disabilities.

Financing Home Accessibility Modifications (Center for Accessible Housing, North Carolina State University, Box 8613, Raleigh, NC 27695, tel: 919-515-3082). This publication identifies state and local sources of financial assistance for homeowners (or tenants) who need to make modifications in their homes.

GE Answer Center (9500 Williamsburg Plaza, Louisville, KY 40222, tel: 800-626-2000). The Center, which is open twenty-four hours a day, seven days a week, offers assistance to individuals with disabilities as well as the general public. They offer two free brochures, "Appliance Help for Those with Special Needs," and "Basic Kitchen Planning for the Physically Handicapped."

National Association of Home Builders (NAHB) (National Research Center, Economics and Policy Analysis Division, 400 Prince George's Boulevard, Upper Marlboro, MD 20772, tel: 301-249-4000). The Research Center produces publications and provides training on housing and special needs. A publication entitled "Homes for a Lifetime" includes an accessibility checklist, financing options, and recommendations for working with builders and remodelers.

National Kitchen and Bath Association (687 Willow Grove Street, Hackettstown, NJ 07840, tel: 908-852-0033). The Association produces a technical manual of barrier-free planning and has directories of certified designers and planners.

Travel

ACCESS: The Foundation for Accessibility by the Disabled (P.O. Box 356, Malverne, NY 11565, tel: 516-887-5798). ACCESS is a clearinghouse for travel services and information on accessibility for the physically disabled. They publish monographs pertaining to travel and accessibility, and will assist in finding resources and services for individuals and corporations.

Directory of Travel Agencies for the Disabled. (Written by Helen Hecker, published by Twin Peaks Press, P.O. Box 129, Vancouver, WA 98666-0129). This directory lists travel agents who specialize in arranging travel plans for people with disabilities.

The Disability Bookshop (P.O. Box 129, Vancouver, WA 98666, tel: 800-637-2256). The Disability Bookshop has an extensive list of books for disabled travelers, dealing with such topics as accessibility, travel agencies, accessible van rentals, medical resources, air travel, and guides to national parks.

Information for Handicapped Travelers (available free of charge from the National Library Service for the Blind and Physically Handicapped, 1291 Taylor Street, N.W., Washington, DC 20542, tel: 800-424-8567; 202-707-5100). A booklet providing information about travel agents, transportation, and information centers for individuals with disabilities.

Project Action (Internet: www.projectaction.org). Maintains a database on its web site of information about the availability of accessible transportation anywhere in the United States. Users can highlight the state and city they plan to visit and view all transportation services available to them. The database also includes travel agencies specializing in travel arrangements for people with disabilities.

Society for the Advancement of Travel for the Handicapped (SATH) (347 Fifth Avenue, Suite 610, New York, NY 10016, tel: 212-447-7284). SATH is a nonprofit organization that acts as a clearinghouse for accessible tourism information and is in contact with organization in many countries to promote the development of facilities for disabled people. SATH publishes a quarterly magazine, "Access to Travel."

Travel for the Disabled: A Handbook of Travel Resources and 500 Worldwide Access Guides. (Written by Helen Hecker, published by Twin Peaks Press, P.O. Box 129, Vancouver, WA 98666, tel: 800-637-2256). The handbook provides information for disabled travelers about accessibility.

Travel Industry and Disabled Exchange (TIDE) (5435 Donna Avenue, Tarzana, CA 91356, tel: 818-343-6339). The Exchange assists disabled individuals to travel throughout the world. A quarterly newsletter is available to members.

Travel Information Service (Moss Rehabilitation Hospital, 1200 West Tabor Road, Philadelphia, PA 19141, tel: 456-4603). The Service provides information and referrals for people with disabilities.

Travelin' Talk (P.O. Box 3534, Clarksville, TN 37043, tel: 615-552-6670). A network of more than one thousand people and organizations around the world who are willing to provide assistance to travelers with disabilities and share their knowledge about the areas in which they live. Travelin' Talk publishes a newsletter by the same name and has an extensive resource directory.

The Wheelchair Traveler (Accent on Living, P.O. Box 700, Bloomington, IL 61702, tel: 309-378-2961). A directory that provides ratings of hotels and motels in the United States.

Wilderness Inquiry (1313 5th Street, S.E., Box 84, Minneapolis, MN 55414, tel: 800-728-0719; 612-379-3858). Wilderness Inquiry sponsors trips into the wilderness for people with disabilities or chronic conditions.

Visual Impairment

Canadian National Institute for the Blind (CNIB) (1931 Bayview Avenue, Toronto, Ontario M4G 4C8, Canada, tel: 416-480-7580). The Institute provides counseling and rehabilitation services for Canadians with any degree of functional visual impairment. They offer public information literature and operate resource and technology centers. The national office has a list of provincial and local CNIB offices.

The Lighthouse Low Vision Products Consumer Catalog (36-20 Northern Boulevard, Long Island City, NY 11101, tel: 800-829-0500). This large-print catalog offers a wide range of products designed to help people with impaired vision.

The Library of Congress, Division for the Blind and Physically Handicapped (1291 Taylor Street, N.W., Washington, DC 20542, tel: 800-424-8567; 800-424-9100; for application: 202-287-5100). The Library Service provides free talking book equipment on loan as well as a full range of recorded books for individuals with disabilities or visual impairment. It also provides a variety of free library services through one hundred forty cooperating libraries.

Living with Low Vision: A Resource Guide for People with Sight Loss. (Published by Resources for Rehabilitation, 33 Bedford Street, Suite 19A, Lexington, MA 02173, tel: 617-862-6455). A comprehensive directory designed to help individuals with impaired vision to locate the products and services they need in order to remain independent.

Products for People with Vision Impairment Catalog. (American Foundation
for the Blind Product Center, P.O. Box 7044, 100 Enterprise Place, Dover,
DE 19903, tel: 800-829-0500). The Catalog is available in standard print
and audiocassette. Inserts from Kalb.
Recording for the Blind, Inc., 20 Roszel Road, Princeton, NJ 08540; (609)
452-0606.

Disease-Modifying Therapies and Patient Assistance Programs

Shared Solutions®

Shared Solutions® is a program sponsored by Teva, Neuroscience, the makers of
Copaxone® and is a free program that is designed to help people with MS, their
families and their care givers. The Shared Solutions® service is individually tailored to the patient using the collective knowledge of leading medical experts
in the field of MS, including nurses. The program aims to help MS patients
overcome the challenges of living with the disease and is also open to patients
who are not receiving Copaxone® therapy. The support services offered by the
Shared Solutions® program include a telephone service where trained professionals, such as nurses, can be reached for advice such as injection administration
tips and information regarding Copaxone® therapy. Shared Solutions® also
organizes events including live discussions and educational programs and help
with reimbursement issues. The program also provides a MS-focused website
along with downloadable resources. Shared Solutions nurses are encouraged
to MS certified and are encouraged to sustain continuing education and information related to their field of expertise. Certain regions of North America
now have specialist nurses to provide injection training in patients' homes.

Avonex Services®

Avonex Services is a new program sponsored by Biogen, makers of Avonex®.
The service is a mentor and advocate program which allows patients to share
their MS and Avonex® experiences with others. The program provides information on reimbursement issues and offers nursing and personal support via
telephone or one-to-one contact within the patient's own home and the provision
of educational materials. The program also allows MS patients to search for, or
become, a MS mentor that helps and supports other MS sufferers by sharing their
experiences on getting started on treatment, choosing a physician, and managing
symptoms. Avonex Services also provides a platform for patients to make an impact
by becoming an advocate and a forum for sharing their personal experiences with
others and for posting MS events.

MS Lifelines™

MS Lifelines is a program sponsored by EMD Serono, the makers of Rebif®. This program provides patient education in MS through a number of services including: facts, tips and support provided by healthcare professionals, including nurses, for patients receiving Rebif® treatment. MS Lifelines™ also provides a range of educational materials such as booklets concerning the disease and information regarding Rebif® therapy. Members can have access to 'ambassadors' (people living well with MS), which is an important aspect of patient-support programs as it enables patients to have continued hope in coming to terms with and coping with MS. Members of the program can also have live discussions via the web or over the telephone, providing help and support to the patient. Rebif® nurses are assigned to train patients and families with injection therapy and techniques, and the nurse will follow them until they can assume more responsibility for self-management. Rebif field nurses are MS specialists and provide injection training and personal assistance to patients and families beginning or sustaining MS therapy. Lifelines nurses and field nurses are encouraged to sit for the specialist examination as well as to attend ongoing nurse education programs.

BETA Nurse/MS Pathways

The Betaseron Education, Training and Assistance (BETA) Nurse/MS Pathways (MSP) program is sponsored by Berlex, the makers of Betaseron®. The BETA Nurse program is unique in that it is a wholly nurse-coordinated service, with a total of 78 specialist nurses enrolled to date. This individual service provides support to MS patients taking Betaseron®, and is also open to patients not receiving Betaseron® therapy. The service is run by specialist MS certified nurses throughout the US known as 'BETA nurses'. Although the BETA Nurse program is specifically centered on the MS patient, the program also offers unique opportunities for the nurse, and provides an atypical nursing career. The program provides nurses with at least 2 months of internal training, after which the nurse (paired with a mentor) will work with MS patients in the home setting or at the BETA center. BETA Nurses are also encouraged to sit for the IOMSN examinationss within 2 years of starting the program.

BETA nurses provide support to MS patients in a number of ways, both in person (home visits or at one of the specialist BETA centers) and via telephone, and all patients are offered the same regular contacts. Providing a regular contact that can provide support in the home is an important factor of patient care, as some patients may find traveling to the hospital or center difficult. This becomes increasingly important if the patient has impaired mobility.[11] The BETA Nurse will initiate telephone counseling and training with the patient, where the nurse provides instruction on the appropriate injection techniques. The BETA Nurse will provide consistent follow-up and will record the patient's progress with therapy. This will include the monitoring of adverse events and tolerance to treatment over time. Additional services offered by the program, and advocated by the BETA Nurse include: invitations to bimonthly seminars that cover educational issues, a platform to share personal experiences with other MS patients, listings of local events and a newsroom service where patients are able to view the latest developments in MS online and information and help regarding reimbursement. The BETA Nurse program has been one of the most successful nurse-coordinated services, and as such, several elements of the program have been incorporated into other support programs.

TABLE A

The Food and Drug Administration Approved Disease-Modifying Therapies Currently Available for Multiple Sclerosis

Drug (tradename)	Manufacturer	Class of Agent	Approved Indication	Mode of Administration	Dosing Frequency
IFN-β-1a (Rebif®)	EMD Serono Rockland, MA	Type I IFN	RRMS For the reduction in the frequency of exacerbations and to delay the accumulation of physical disability	0.5/0.2 mL prefilled syringe for s.c. injection (22/44 mcg IFN)	3 times a week, at least 48 hours apart
IFN-β-1a (Avonex®)	Biogen IDEC Inc, Cambridge, MA	Type I IFN	RRMS For the reduction in the frequency of exacerbations and to delay the accumulation of physical disability	0.5 mL prefilled syringe for IM injection (30 mcg IFN)	Once a week
IFN-β-1b (Betaseron®)	Berlex Laboratories, Wayne, NJ	Type I IFN	RRMS For the reduction in the frequency of clinical exacerbations	Sterile lyophilized powder in 3 mL vials, for 1 mL SC injection (8 MIU/mL IFN)	Every other day
Glatiramer acetate (Copaxone®)	Teva Neuroscience, Kansas City, MO	Co-polymer I	RRMS For the reduction of frequency of relapses in ambulatory patients who have had at least two relapses in the preceding 2 years before initiation of therapy	0.1 mL solution for s.c. injection (20 mg glatiramer acetate)	Daily

Mitoxantrone (Novantrone®)	EMD Serono Rockland, MA	Antitumor antibiotic	Worsening RRMS PRMS SPMS For the reduction in the frequency of clinical relapses and to delay the accumulation of neurologic disability	12 mg/m^2 given as 5 to 15 IV infusions	Every 3 months
Natalizumab (Tysabri®)	Biogen IDEC Inc, Cambridge, MA	Monoclonal antibody	RRMS: recommended for patients who have had an inadequate response to, or are unable to tolerate, alternate MS therapies To be used as a monotherapy only For the reduction in the frequency of clinical exacerbations and to delay the accumulation of physical disability	15 mL dose (300 mg natalizumab) IV infusion	Every 4 weeks

IFN=interferon; RR=relapsing remitting; MS=multiple sclerosis; PR=progressive relapsing; s.c.=subcutaneous; SP=secondary progressive; IM=intramuscular; IV=intravenous.

TABLE B

Overview of Patient Assistance Programs Currently Available for Multiple Sclerosis Patients

Company	Product	Nurse Program	Description	Number of Nurses/Patients	Services Offered	Web Links
Berlex	Interferon β-1b (Beta-seron®)	BETA Nurse MS Pathways	Part of the BETA (Beta-seron Education, Training and Assistance) nurse program, this is a personalized support program that connects people with MS who are starting on Betaseron® (interferon beta-1b) for s.c. injection with a dedicated MS nurse specialist. Berlex created the B.E.T.A. nurse program in May 2002	50 MS nurse specialists	o Education on managing MS o Training o Assistance through wphone calls o Betanurse – real time website	www.betanurses.com www.mspathways.com
Biogen /Idec	Interferon β-1a (Avonex®)	Mentor training	Offers a Mentor and Advocate program – training people with experience of MS who want to be of assistance	N/A	o Personal training on injections by a qualified nurse o An Avonex® Case Manager, knowledgeable about MS and Avonex®	http://www.avonex.com/msavProject/avonexportal/_baseurl/threeColLayout/SCSRepository/en_US/avonex/home/avonex-services/index.xml

EMD Serono	Interferon β-1a (Rebif®)	MS Lifelines	Serono recently launched a team of nurse educators who are dedicated to MS and available to provide education and in-home injection training to Rebif® patients	N/A	o Online lifelines website with up to date MS information o Manned phone line for help and information	http://www.mslifelines.com/index.jsp
TEVA Neuroscience	Glatiramer acetate (Copaxone®)	Shared Solutions® MSWatch®	A voluntary, free program designed to help people with MS, their families and their caregivers confront and manage the challenges of MS This is one of the largest online communities for all people with MS and their care partners	N/A	o A series of monthly teleconferences and seminars covering the latest issues and developments in MS o Comprehensive network of resources to help patients get started with Copaxone® o Free phone line 12 hrs a day to a trained professional o Educational seminars	http://www.mswatch.com/

Index